THE HOSPITAL EXECUTIVE'S GUIDE TO EMERGENCY DEPARTMENT MANAGEMENT

KIRK B. JENSEN, MD, MBA, FACEP

DANIEL G. KIRKPATRICK, MHA, FACHE

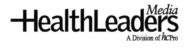

HealthLeaders *Media*
A Division of *hc*Pro

+HCPro

The Hospital Executive's Guide to Emergency Department Management is published by HCPro, Inc.

Copyright © 2010 HCPro, Inc.

All rights reserved. Printed in the United States of America.   5   4   3   2

ISBN: 978-1-60146-742-3

Kirk B. Jensen, MD, MBA, FACEP, Author   Mike Mirabello, Senior Graphic Artist
Daniel G. Kirkpatrick, MHA, FACHE, Author   Amanda Donaldson, Copyeditor
Carrie Vaughan, Editor   Sada Preisch, Proofreader
Rick Johnson, Executive Editor   Matt Sharpe, Production Supervisor
Matt Cann, Group Publisher   Susan Darbyshire, Art Director
Doug Ponte, Cover Designer   Jean St. Pierre, Senior Director of Operations

Advice given is general. Readers should consult professional counsel for specific legal, ethical, or clinical questions. Arrangements can be made for quantity discounts. For more information, contact:

HCPro, Inc.
75 Sylvan Street, Suite A-101
Danvers, MA 01923
Telephone: 800/650-6787 or 781/639-1872
Fax: 800/639-8511
E-mail: *customerservice@hcpro.com*

Visit HCPro online at: *www.hcpro.com* and *www.hcmarketplace.com*

Rev. 09/2011
49582

Contents

Chapter 7: Culture and Change Management **157**

Chapter 8: Patient Safety and Risk Reduction **171**

Chapter 9: The Role and Necessity of the Dashboard **191**

Chapter 10: Physician Compensation: Productivity-Based Systems **203**

About the Authors

Kirk B. Jensen, MD, MBA, FACEP

Kirk B. Jensen, MD, MBA, FACEP, has spent more than 20 years in emergency medicine management and clinical care. He is board certified in emergency medicine and the chief medical officer of BestPractices, Inc., an emergency medicine leadership and staffing practice based in Fairfax, VA. Jensen is one of the most widely respected experts in patient safety, performance improvement, and patient flow, and he has developed some of the most innovative solutions in emergency medicine.

Jensen is directly responsible for the coaching, mentoring, and career development of medical directors for BestPractices. He also serves as a medical director for The Studer Group, an international outcomes-based healthcare organization, in Gulf Breeze, FL, that assists hospitals in improving clinical and operations results.

Jensen has been on the faculty of the Institute for Healthcare Improvement (IHI) since 1998 and has coached more than 300 emergency departments (ED) through the process of improving operations and clinical services. He chaired the IHI's Learning and Innovation Communities on *Operational and Clinical Improvement in the Emergency Department* and *Improving Flow Through the Acute Care Setting*, and he currently leads the innovative seminars *Cracking the Code to*

Hospital-wide Patient Flow and *Perfecting Emergency Department Operations.* His other accomplishments include:

- Leading two hospitals to national benchmark standards in ED operations and efficiency, while serving as medical director and chair of the ED

- Implementing procedures that achieved national recognition for Nash General Hospital in Rocky Mount, NC, as it was designated a "Best Practice Clinical Site" by the Emergency Nurses Association in 1999

- Serving as a certified MedTeams instructor

- Sitting on the expert panel and site examination team for Urgent Matters, a Robert Wood Johnson Foundation Initiative focusing on reducing ED crowding

- Coauthoring the 2007 Hamilton Award–winning book *Leadership for Smooth Patient Flow* and the 2009 book *Hardwiring Flow*

- Teaching at the American College of Emergency Physicians Directors Academy, leading ED directors through process improvements in patient flow, error reduction, and managing change

Jensen holds a bachelor's degree in biology from the University of Illinois in Champaign and a medical degree from the University of Illinois in Chicago. He completed his residency in emergency medicine at the University of Chicago and earned an MBA from the University of Tennessee in Knoxville. He recently completed the Lean for Healthcare course at the University of Tennessee Center for Executive Education.

Daniel G. Kirkpatrick, MHA, FACHE

Daniel G. Kirkpatrick, MHA, FACHE, has more than 28 years of healthcare management experience in consulting, staff, and administrator roles, and he leads practice operations at BestPractices, Inc., an emergency medicine leadership and staffing practice based in Fairfax, VA. Kirkpatrick has extensive consulting experience helping group practices and hospitals in meeting their operational and financial goals, as well as enhancing their service, leadership, safety, and sustainability performance. Previously, he worked in public accounting; held administrative roles in hospitals including for-profit, nonprofit, specialty medical-surgical, and behavioral health entities; and provided extensive practice management for medical practices, including primary care, specialty, and hospital-based entities. This experience provided him knowledge of and sensitivity to the complex issues confronting healthcare providers.

Kirkpatrick holds a BA in psychology from the College of Wooster in Ohio and an MHA from Ohio State University. He and his wife and children live in eastern North Carolina.

Acknowledgments

I've been privileged to have been raised by parents who have dedicated their lives to helping others and have instilled in me and my siblings the values of integrity, compassion, respect, and "principles over personalities." Thanks, Mom and Dad, for setting the bar high and challenging us to stay above it!

I'm clearly indebted to Kirk Jensen for offering me the opportunity to collaborate on this book, and for his selfless mentoring and patience. A special thanks to Thom Mayer for demonstrating tactical wisdom and relentless optimism, which are great qualities in emergency medicine.

The steadfast support, understanding, and patience of a loving wife cannot be overstated and were essential as I pursued this project—thanks, Allison, for always being there for me and thanks to my kids for keeping me honest and keeping me young.

A special thanks to my partners in Four Guys—truer friends don't exist.

Daniel G. Kirkpatrick, MHA, FACHE

The Hospital Executive's Guide to Emergency Department Management

This book is the result of our combined efforts, knowledge, and experience on the subject of ED management. Our years of clinical practice, mentoring, partnering with, and learning from our client hospitals and hospital teams across the country have contributed to our current understanding of leadership, management, teamwork, patient flow, and safety, and its importance in the lives of our patients, co-workers, and clients.

Many individuals and organizations have contributed to our evolving understanding of how to improve ED operations and management. BestPractices, Inc., the Institute for Healthcare Improvement, Associates in Process Improvement, Lean For Healthcare, and The Studer Group have all provided opportunities to learn, grow, share, and implement positive and productive change. We would like to acknowledge Eric Minkove, Thom Mayer, Kevin Nolan, Jody Crane, and Chuck Noon for their interest and support in our quest.

Robert Milks was of great help in producing and editing the manuscript. Special thanks to Ashley Jones for her contributions to the work.

I would like to thank my co-author Dan for his friendship and collaboration on this book. I want to acknowledge my parents, Earl and Naomi, who as the parents of eight children first introduced me to the importance of management and organization. My sons Christopher and Michael are constant reminders of what is truly important in life. To my wife Karen, thank you for cutting a wide berth as I worked long hours on yet another project.

Kirk B. Jensen, MD, MBA, FACEP

Introduction:
Why the ED Matters

Acute care settings are often plagued with waits, delays, and dissatisfaction. Nowhere is this more observable and its impact more palpable than in hospital emergency departments (ED). Hospitals are increasingly being challenged to address ED service and quality. A recent report from the Institute of Medicine, *Hospital-Based Emergency Care: At the Breaking Point,* has focused significant attention on this topic. EDs are busy places and only getting busier, and when patients, information, and materials do not flow through the ED in a timely and efficient way, patient safety, patient and staff satisfaction, and hospital bottom lines can all be negatively affected.

This book outlines and defines key challenges, opportunities, and constraints within the ED. We draw lessons from operations and service management and lessons grounded in extensive experience in the real world. We describe the key strategies and best practices that have been developed not only to improve your department but to optimize it. In doing so, we define key barriers and bottlenecks preventing great patient care and we offer solutions to these problems. This book focuses on the following four key drivers affecting ED service and performance:

1. Leadership

2. Service operations

3. The effective use of data

4. Making the right diagnosis and applying the right treatment

Every healthcare leader wants his or her hospital to be successful in a competitive marketplace while providing services that its community requires. An emergency department that works can be a distinctive service that helps leaders accomplish both missions. But many, if not most, healthcare leaders feel they have not achieved this goal in their ED. This is not a result of disinterest or a lack of trying. Most hospital executives are fully aware that the ED is now the front door to their healthcare facility, with 50%–70%[1] of hospital admissions arriving through the ED. While some hospital executives may neither like nor want this state of affairs, most understand it is a condition of healthcare today. That's why many have embedded in the hospital's core mission and strategic plan a desire to have a department that they are not only proud of but that they would be willing to visit as a patient or family member of a patient. However, quality, safety, and service can seem fleeting: there for one minute, one day, one shift, or one patient, and then gone the next, seemingly without cause or explanation.

EDs are complex, often chaotic environments—microsystems that can challenge even the best of leaders. EDs contribute to many important apsects of the hospital, such as patient and employee satisfaction, patient safety, risk reduction, evidence-based outcomes, and even profitability. Therefore, it is imperative for healthcare executives to build processes that can stabilize the ED's performance in the areas of quality, safety, and service. The ED can be, and should be, an asset that gives healthcare systems a substantial service advantage and competitive edge.

Why Improvement Is Necessary

Emergency medicine is a professional and business service that often involves out-sourced contract services. But it is only as good as the service it provides—or is *perceived* to provide. Because the ED is the front door of the hospital and accounts for such a large part of hospital admissions, how the department is viewed has a direct impact on how the hospital itself is perceived by the community. A bad patient experience in the ED has a way of making itself known to administration, the board of trustees, and the public. Thus, ensuring that things run smoothly and professionally in the ED is in the hospital executive's best interest.

Traditionally, the nursing management team has run the ED with input from the ED physician group. Nursing staff members are more often than not hospital employees. The physicians may be employed directly by the hospital; however, many hospitals contract with staffing groups or companies to provide physician and management services. A hospital board and administrator have several options when deciding how their emergency care center will be staffed—from small, independent, physician-owned groups to large, nationwide staffing companies. These groups compete on the basis of services provided, economics, and the targeted needs of each hospital.

Historically, hospitals have accepted "good enough" as satisfactory performance from their EDs. But a "gentleman's C" may no longer be a passing grade, thanks to the baby boomer generation. As this population ages, emphasis will increasingly be placed on the issues of patient safety and satisfaction, risk reduction, timeliness of care, and a satisfied medical staff.

The nature of the problem

On March 31, 2003, the General Accounting Office (GAO) issued a report, *Hospital Emergency Departments: Crowded Conditions Vary among Hospitals and Communities*, warning that the nation's EDs are under strain and that systemwide change is needed to correct the problems.[2] The 2009 Report, *Hospital Emergency Departments: Crowding Continues To Occur, and Some Patients Wait Longer than Recommended Time Frames* reaffirms those findings.[3] In a survey of 2,000 hospitals, the GAO found that two-thirds of all EDs diverted ambulances to other hospitals at some point during fiscal year 2001. One-third of the hospitals boarded about 75% of their patients in the ED for two or more hours in the previous year, while three-fourths of hospitals experienced some form of boarding.

Both reports suggested that financial pressures lead hospitals to limit capacity, making it difficult for them to meet periodic spikes in demand for inpatient beds. Those same pressures also lead to competition between ED admissions and scheduled admissions, such as surgery patients, who are generally considered more profitable. Herein lies a significant dilemma. If the more profitable cases are not served, less money is available to help meet the space, staffing, and equipment needs of the less profitable cases. Hospital officials indicated that emergency patients are less profitable because a larger proportion of emergency admissions are for patients who self-pay (including the uninsured) and generally provide lower reimbursement, the study found.

While the federal government has realized that there is a serious problem in EDs and is funding a prominent Institute of Medicine agency to look into that problem, don't expect tangible help in the foreseeable future. EDs need do to what they can to solve the problems of overcrowding and diversion themselves. What do we have control over and what can we do? Consider some myths and realities:

Myth 1: Managed care has decreased ED volume.
Reality: From 1996 to 2006, ED utilization rose by 32%.

Myth 2: ED diversion and boarding patients is a regional phenomenon.
Reality: 75% of all hospitals divert patients.

Myth 3: Nonurgent ED volume has risen dramatically.
Reality: Nonurgent volume has remained stable, while critical-care volume has risen 50% in the past 10 years.[4]

Although all of these myths shape the perceptions and operations of EDs, it is myth 3—that there are too many patients in the ED who do not belong there—that is the most pervasive and persistent. Everyone from the hospital administrator to the average person on the street seems to think EDs are overcrowded because too many patients are treated there who should be treated somewhere else. This perception raises two points:

- Since the federal government, through the Emergency Medical Treatment and Active Labor Act of 1986 (EMTALA), requires that every patient in an ED be examined and stabilized, what else are EDs expected or able to do for patients?

- Studies show that walk-in volume is not an independent predictor of diversion. Michael J. Schull, MD, for example, found that diversion had nothing to do with walk-in flow.[5] It had everything to do with how many patients were being boarded in the ED. Staff members in the ED certainly feel overworked or overwhelmed because of the volume of walk-ins, but that is not what causes diversion. Diversion is not a walk-in problem. ED diversion is an inpatient access problem.

A multitude of factors are responsible for crowding, such as:

- ED patients are sicker, but getting patients admitted is more difficult than ever. Hospitals are trying to run at close to 100% occupancy—a factory model where everybody is busy all the time and there is seldom unused capacity. Hospitals aim at maximizing revenues, but without surge or backup capacity, inpatient admissions from the ED can be delayed, resulting in decreased patient satisfaction and other service and safety problems.

- There aren't enough nurses to meet patient demand. The severe nursing shortage is causing nurses to be overloaded. In addition, The Joint Commission has found that this overloading causes 25% of all medical errors.[6]

- Lack of access to on-call specialists can delay care and slow down the admission process. Because EMTALA requires hospitals to accept all cases and transfers requiring a higher level of care, specialists are effectively on call for an entire state or region.

- Many patients using the ED, such as the uninsured, have little or no alternative for medical care. The ED offers these patients high-quality care, access to every diagnostic test the hospital offers, and guaranteed treatment without any up-front cost. These patients will continue to use the ED as their primary care provider until a better system is found.

All of these factors contribute to problems ranging from difficulties with staffing and resources to compromises in patient care and safety.

A Quest for Excellence

The current state of the American healthcare system is obviously a central issue, and national attention is focused on the core issues of patient satisfaction; patient safety; risk reduction; process improvement; risk management; and employee recruitment, retention, and satisfaction. Not surprisingly, these topics have caught the attention of many upper-level hospital administrators as well. Many hospital leaders have turned to industry experts in an effort to integrate safety and satisfaction programs from other fields (such as the aerospace industry and nuclear power facilities) into the hospital and ED setting. The problem (or potential, depending on your point of view) lies in the disparity between the high level of interest in these core issues and the ability to effectively implement and sustain the solutions.

Even in hospitals and EDs where the required competencies are available, the ability to effectively integrate them into a functioning and effective program may not exist.

This book is designed to solve specific problems encountered in an often over-burdened and inefficient ED. Our goal is to create unique and replicable processes that ensure increased productivity, safety, and patient satisfaction. And we have not just a goal, but a vision that:

- Every ED will be noted for its commitment to quality and excellence and offer the finest possible service in emergency physician leadership, management, clinical care, patient satisfaction, and patient safety to not only patients but also to hospitals, physicians, and medical staffs

- Every patient will experience and receive this care

- Every healthcare worker (many of them heroes already) will get to practice in this type of environment and facility

The process of elevating the game of your ED to this level and then sustaining that performance is a worthy challenge, one with tremendous potential to improve patient care and safety, as well as to provide returns to the bottom line. We'll define the key operational tools and techniques that have the power to turn every ED into a state-of-the-art practice.

References

1. Centers for Disease Control and Prevention, National Center for Health Care Statistics. "National Hospital Ambulatory Medical Care Survey: 2006 Emergency Department Summary," No. 7, August 6, 2006.

2. United States Government Accounting Office. Hospital Emergency Departments: Crowded Conditions Vary among Hospitals and Communities, 2003.

3. United States Government Accounting Office. Hospital Emergency Departments: Crowding Continues To Occur, and Some Patients Wait Longer than Recommended Time Frames, 2009.

4. Centers for Disease Control and Prevention, National Center for Health Care Statistics. "National Hospital Ambulatory Medical Care Survey: 2006 Emergency Department Summary," No. 7, August 6, 2006.

5. Schull, M.J., Lazier, K., Vermeulen, M., Mawhinney, S., and Morrison, L.J. 2003a. "Emergency Department Contributors of Ambulance Diversion: A Quantitative Analysis." *Annals of Emergency Medicine* 41 (4): 467–76.

6. Aiken, L.H., Clark, S.P., Sloane, D.M., Sochalski, J., Silber, J.H. Hospital Nurse Staffing and Patient Mortality, Nurse Burnout, and Job Dissatisfaction. *JAMA.* 2002;288:1987–1193.

A Design for Operational Excellence

Organizations should implement a comprehensive design for ED patient flow, services, and operations to ensure their ED provides every patient the finest clinical care in a safe environment and meets or exceeds patient, staff, and physician satisfaction goals. We've identified eight key components that should be included in this design.

Key Components

Before you can devise a plan for improving an ED, you must have a reasonable idea of what you're getting into, and to obtain that requires drawing an accurate picture of what the current department is like.

Making the right ED diagnosis

A critical first step is to carry out an environmental assessment to determine what the strengths and weaknesses of the department are, what areas need to be fixed immediately, and what areas require planned long-term change for future payoff.

Using information gathered during the assessment, along with input from the on-site team, the project leader should sort the ED into one of six categories (see Figure 1.1) and develop a treatment plan.

FIGURE 1.1

A DIAGNOSTIC MODEL

1. **A Major Project**: seriously deficient in all major areas; requires intensive work; success is not assured

2. **A Complete Turnaround**: requires significant investment of effort and time on the part of the management team due to serious deficiencies in staffing, operations, and leadership

3. **A Fixer-Upper**: requires upgrading in just one or perhaps two of the core elements (staffing, operations, or leadership)

4. **Basic Rebranding and Realignment**: requires moderate upgrade in one or two of the major components of the ED program

5. **Leadership Development**: the major deficiency is in leadership; requires upgrading, coaching, or recruiting the necessary leadership

6. **Business as Usual**: "staying the course"—a well-run facility; requires continuing and maintaining the current model

---

The Hospital Executive's Guide to Emergency Department Management

The assessment component should include the following three basic steps:

1. Review of key documents

    -   Physician and nurse schedules

    -   Patient volume, variation, and trends

    -   Cycle times for patient flow, subprocesses, and ancillary services

    -   Patient satisfaction survey results (both inpatient and ED)

    -   Evaluation and management coding broken down by payer and trended over time

    -   Review of any previous ED studies (The Joint Commission, risk management, internal review and strategic plan, consulting reports)

    -   Organizational chart and administrative architecture

2. A two-day on-site operations assessment

    -   Interview with all key participants

    -   Interview with representative samples of all "service-line" people who provide direct patient care

– Direct observation of patient flow

– Direct observation of team interactions

3. Formulation of an action plan and selection of performance improvement teams

Recruiting, credentialing, and retaining your team

We cannot overemphasize how critical recruiting, credentialing, and retention are in establishing a smoothly running ED. Hiring correctly is a cornerstone of quality, safety, and service. Indeed, the most important part of optimizing an ED's development and operational design is recruiting and employing the requisite professional staff. Yet hiring the right people is easier said than done. You may have to use many approaches in selecting medical professionals, such as:

• Interviewing and assessing those professionals already on-site

• Use of direct mail

• Telemarketing and cold calling

• Advertising

• Word-of-mouth advertising

• Use of professional recruiting firms

• Interaction with various training and professional programs

It is an arduous process with no guarantee of immediate success. It requires an effective, reliable way to screen for and select the desired attributes. You must rely on professional training, references, personal interviews—and a bit of luck.

Once you've chosen the appropriate medical professional, and the job offer has been accepted and secured, the next step is to credential the physician or midlevel provider for hospital privileges as quickly and seamlessly as possible. This process is also labor intensive, requiring coordination by the hospital credentialing service, the group's credentialing staff, and the medical professional.

The higher goals are to carefully select highly trained and motivated professionals, provide a setting of support, and align their goals with the strategic objectives of the hospital, the nursing staff, the medical staff, and the community.

Leadership selection and development

Equally critical in the success of any ED is selecting and developing effective medical leadership. Because the medical director is the most influential physician employee in the ED contract group, the administration must carefully select, coach, and mentor that individual. Similarly, the ED nurse manager or director is the most prominent nursing employee in the department, so administrators should just as carefully select, coach, and mentor that person as well. If you want to succeed in your mission of effectively serving the hospital and its patients, the director is critical to the mission. The director acts as the coach and general manager of the "service franchise." To enable the director to effectively fulfill that role, you must assess, reinforce, and enhance his or her leadership and change-management skills.

To support your director, you should employ a teaching, coaching, and mentoring process. One recommendation is enrolling the director in a leadership institute for further leadership development as well as collaboration with peers. As a leader and manager, you should use a balanced scorecard format to continually monitor and evaluate the department and the director's performance.

This approach focuses on four areas: safety, service, sustainability, and staff. The director and the team must achieve measurable success in all four quadrants to optimize patient flow and service within the ED. In using the balanced scorecard, you set goals and metrics. Weekly conference calls and quarterly ED practice reviews help implement the scorecard and keep it in play.

Patient flow and operations management

Flow can be defined as the movement of people and materials through a service system. In working to improve flow, hospitals apply strategies developed both within and outside the healthcare industry. Flow is not unique to healthcare, but it is an important element of many service and industrial processes. We define patient flow in the ED as the movement of patients from the time they enter the department until the time they are released or are admitted to the hospital, and if they are admitted, then until the time they are discharged from the ED to the floor. The following are the nine key principles in making patient management more efficient and effective:

1. Match capacity to demand

2. Monitor patient flow in real time

3. Help shape demand

4. Manage, reduce, or eliminate variability

5. Reduce waste (anything that does not add value to the service or to the encounter)

6. Forecast and predict demand for services

7. Understand the implications and insights of queuing and queuing theory

8. Understand the implications and insights of the Theory of Constraints

9. Appreciate that the ED is part of a system

The process of improving patient flow begins with analyzing all the relevant metrics and reviewing all the previous studies of patient flow. It continues with the two-day, hands-on operational assessment we described earlier. The management and operational team should then be guided, coached, and mentored by establishing and coaching performance improvement teams through the production and execution of a process-improvement task matrix.

Performance improvement teams play a vital role in the development of hospital processes and relationships. Any critical-care area, such as the ED or the department of surgery, can develop an "us versus the world" mentality. With their particular needs and demands for special skills, these departments commonly become isolated, working as silos. Yet this mentality is counterproductive to smoothing flow throughout the unit and integrating flow with the rest of the hospital. Since more than half of the admissions coming into any hospital arrive through the ED, this integration is important. With coaching and process-improvement strategies in place, the ED staff can move beyond its silo and help significantly increase the efficiency of the hospital as a whole.

Customer service and survival skills

Patient satisfaction and excellent customer service are critical attributes of high-performance EDs. Patients, medical staffs, and hospital administrators have come to value satisfaction and service as defining features of quality healthcare. Two factors are converging that will likely make the provision of satisfactory service an even stronger driver in healthcare: the fact that consumer culture continues to infiltrate the medical world, and the aging of the baby boomer generation. ED staff members should be trained in these aspects of healthcare. Tools such as our Survival Skills© training course can be used as part of the on-boarding process.

Developed during the past 10 years, the course focuses on the needs of healthcare workers and the attributes and actions necessary to deliver high-quality customer service. Practicing emergency physicians and nurses who are experienced in the realities, limitations, and opportunities present in real-life EDs lead the course. Survival Skills is augmented by the tracking and trending of individualized patient satisfaction scores and targeted and focused individual coaching. Further, each physician should be recruited with customer service skills in mind, and those skills should be monitored by compliment-and-complaint analysis.

Change management

Improvements mean change, and embarking on cultural change can be quite challenging. It requires patience, humor, and tenacity. Physicians and nurses are not always early adopters of change. They are highly intelligent individuals who are trained to be independent and often don't see themselves as part of a possible problem. When you set out to improve your ED, a significant part of your time is going to be spent interacting with physicians, earning their trust, and then obtaining agreement on the vision, mission, values, and goals of the department that coincide with their clinical practices. With the right investments in time, metrics, and communication, you can take major steps toward optimizing any ED.

Success in managing change depends fundamentally on a positive, proactive, and evolving relationship with each partner in the clinical provision of care. In the ED, our partners include the hospital, the medical staff, patients, and physicians and midlevel practitioners. It is crucial to align strategic incentives among each of those partners to ensure that their needs are met to the best extent possible. The best way to meet those needs is to engage our emergency physicians and nurses in an intensive change-management process. This program, which was outlined in the American College of Emergency Physicians white paper on ED operations management, delineates the following five steps:[1]

1. Bring dissatisfaction with the present state into the open and create a sense of urgency

2. Communicate a clear vision of the proposed change

3. Promote participation in the proposed change

4. Communicate clearly

5. Maintain the commitment

Organizational change can seem like navigating through swirling rapids. You find your way through them by a combination of diagnostic assessments, team and leadership development, establishing a common vision, creating an ongoing dialogue, and implementing measures and rewards that monitor the process and promote the envisioned results. Always keep in mind that people support what they help create. If they are with you on the takeoff, they will be with you at the landing.

Building a risk-free ED

The key to successful management of professional liability exposure is not just risk management—which is, after all, dealing with problems after they have occurred—but risk reduction: creating, implementing, and monitoring a system that reduces risk by preventing medical errors from occurring in the ED. To reduce the risk of medical errors, organizations should implement programs that integrate staff education, ongoing Internet training, and continuous monitoring of high-risk areas. With professional liability premiums continuing to rise, establishing a risk-free ED not only enhances patient safety but also frees up clinical practice revenues for rewarding the clinicians who practice in a safe and measured manner.

Having staff members who communicate effectively and work well together for the common goals of safety and excellent service is critical to risk reduction.

We fully embrace the principles of teamwork and training embedded within the discipline of crew-resource management. In all of our EDs, the physicians, midlevel practitioners, and nurses undergo training in teamwork through crew-resource management. As with so many of our programs, we achieve success through education, training, mentoring, and focused repetition. An incentive program rewards and reinforces the desired behaviors.

Billing and collection

Billing and collection are traditionally outsourced. The billing process is complicated, requiring a certain level of tenacity, experience, and expertise. Amounting to approximately 8%–15% of revenue, it is one of the largest expenses after wages. As a staffing company grows, it can consider acquiring or developing an internal billing system as a means to save capital and, in the future, generate new revenue. Each ED should have on-site office staff members responsible and accountable for ensuring that each chart is signed, properly coded, and promptly sent to the billing component. Any holdup in the charting process will have direct ramifications on the flow of revenue. Coding, billing, and collecting are critical to the success of the operation.

Make a Plan and Stick to It

When you set out to evaluate your ED, you should follow a defined, scripted, and sequenced process. For example, the following is the outline of our On-Boarding™ program on how to evaluate and on-board a new ED affiliate:

- The process takes six to 12 months, with the majority of the work occurring within the first 90–120 days

- Significant scheduled points of contact occur in months one, two, three, six, nine, and 12

- Scheduled project milestones in months six and 12 assess actions and progress to date and include a review of progress with the on-site medical director

- Assessment involves the use of a proprietary balanced scorecard approach, key metrics, and multiple sources of feedback

ON-BOARDING™ ASSESSMENT EXAMPLE

During the first 90 to 120 days, there should be three individualized department assessments that result in three corresponding concrete actions tailored to the facility.

Assessment 1: Patient satisfaction

The first assessment is an in-depth examination of the current patient satisfaction tool and its results. After the assessment, we provide our patient satisfaction and customer service training course and survival skills, with emphasis placed on those areas flagged as deficient in the patient satisfaction survey. Because patient satisfaction is an outcome of a system, we enroll all the ED staff members—physicians, nurses, administrative assistants, and support staff members—in the one-day course.

Assessment 2: Operations and patient flow

We carry out a two-day assessment of ED operations and patient flow using our ED Metrics Assessment Intake Tool™. This phase involves a previsit assessment of throughput and operations data and a two-day visit in the department. Activities include interviews with everyone involved in operating a successful ED—lab, x-ray, pharmacy, nursing, and the medical staff and hospital management. The operations assessment also includes several hours of direct observations and analysis during the course of multiple clinical shifts. Resulting from this assessment are a preliminary summary of the findings and plans for development of a six- to 12-month action plan for operational improvements, presented to the medical director and the process improvement team.

Assessment 3: Risk management and patient safety

Finally, we assess risk management, using either a survey previously done by the malpractice carrier or performing our own environmental assessment. This stage culminates with our Creating the Risk-Free ED™ course, a half-day, on-site review of the high-risk, problem-prone areas in emergency medicine (an Internet-based version is also available). Again, because safety and risk management are properties of individual and system performance, all key personnel are enrolled in the course. It includes a session on crew-resource management or teamwork training, as well as an opportunity for the staff to craft local responses to the issues that arise. Web-based risk-management tools, support, and feedback are also utilized.

Optimizing High-Quality Care

If our goal is to optimize high-quality medical care in the ED, taking a look at how we define quality might be useful. In order to do so, we must return to the following five "rights" of medical administration:

1. **The right care:** This topic has been a focus of media attention since Lucian Leape published his first article about it, *Error in Medicine*. *USA Today* published a full-page article, with photos, focusing on medical errors. With more than 6,000 deaths per year in the United States alone attributed to medical errors, providing the right care must be the primary concern.

2. **To the right person:** As the case of Jessica Santillan, the patient who received the wrong heart at Duke University Medical Center, so tragically illustrates, delivering the right care to the right person is of ultimate importance.

3. **At the right time:** The length of stay in an ED is the primary indicator of the quality of care the ED is able to give. When patients wait five hours in the waiting room, the staff members have been stressed for five hours before they even see those patients. More and more, nurses are working a 12-hour shift, and we know that 75% of medical errors made by nurses on a 12-hour shift come in the last few hours, when they are exhausted. Industry studies dating back more than 35 years have proven that spending more than 10 hours on a specific task creates problems with efficiency and effectiveness.[2] Timeliness in the delivery of care must be a high priority.

4. **In the right place:** Delivering care in the right place is critical for an ED. If patients waiting to be admitted occupy 16 of an ED's 17 beds, those patients are not in the right place. If an ED nurse has three critical patients in ED beds and five in the hallway, those patients are not in the right place. In situations such as these, which are common in EDs, the hospital cannot deliver quality care. We must reshape the system to provide the best possible chance for the patient to have a positive outcome.

5. **By the right people.**

The patient experience

The ED should do all it can to make sure that the patient has a satisfactory care experience. This does not mean that we can guarantee outcomes. Historically, we have talked in healthcare about concrete and measurable patient outcomes; we can deliver very good care overall and yet still have adverse outcomes or patients who are highly displeased with their care. Medicine has become a scientific, technically accurate practice, with practitioners well educated in the science of healthcare. Yet the patient often does not get the healing touch that comes with time spent at the bedside. If patients are not satisfied, they will voice their displeasure to a wide audience and seek care elsewhere.

The ED staff's experience

The key to a positive staff experience lies in spending time with the patient and creating a positive environment in which to work. First, a positive environment draws staff members, which in turn contributes to creating more time available for each patient. Originally, religious organizations trained nurses to be nurturers.

Caring for people was the hallmark of the profession. The satisfaction that comes from this experience draws good nurses to the profession and keeps them there. As the nursing profession has evolved, however, nurses are now required to be technical specialists who often have little time to connect with and nurture patients. This has created an environment high in frustration and low in career satisfaction, but the situation can be improved. For example, in one hospital ED, we began with a 33% RN vacancy rate, and nurses were overwhelmed and overworked. One year later, 11 nurses within the hospital system were waiting to come to work in the ED. Changing the environment by training and grooming the staff with a positive attitude transformed the ED for both workers and patients.

Don Berwick, president and founder of the Institute for Healthcare Improvement, makes the point that every systematic process is designed to produce the exact results it does produce. For example, if your patients have been waiting five hours, your system is designed to produce that result. If medical errors occur in 20% of your interventions, your system is set up to produce that error rate. If you have 10 admissions per night sitting on gurneys in the ED hallways or occupying your critical-care beds, your system enables that kind of result. If you want a different outcome, you have to change the system.

References

1. Emergency Department Operations Management: An Information Paper. ACEP. March 2004.

2. Rogers, A.E., Hwang, W.T., Scott, L., Aiken, L., and Dinges, D. The working hours of hospital staff nurses and patient safety. *Health Affairs*. 2004: 23: 202–212.

Leadership

Improving your ED for your patients and staff members will require new ideas. In our experience, most hospitals and departments focus on the quest for ideas to improve the ED. But ideas, while necessary and desirable, are not enough to transform the ED experience on their own. First, organizations must garner a high commitment from senior administrators and a strong will on their part to execute the new processes. It is paramount for organizations to have that leadership throughout all levels of the healthcare team. The process of change has a parallel track: developing leaders throughout the team.

> *There will be challenges. People will find 1,000 ingenious ways to withhold cooperation from a process that they feel is unnecessary or wrong-headed.*
> —John Kotter[1]

Persuading the High Cs

Persuading ED staff members to become enthusiastically involved in improving the department's performance is a major task. But another type of persuasion should come first: convincing the top leadership of the hospital that the project to improve performance is essential and will bring impressive results. Their commitment to the project and its implementation are crucial to the project's success. What we call the "high Cs"—the CEO, chief operating officer, chief medical officer, and chief of emergency medicine, as well as similar officers with commensurate responsibilities in the system—must be brought on board at the beginning. Of course, if the project originates from one of them, then your hospital is already one step ahead.

The following are some reasons this step is so important:

- EDs are part of a set of complex, interdependent microsystems

- One department alone cannot achieve optimized performance for the entire system

- Improving performance in the ED requires high levels of cooperation and integration across multiple disciplines and personnel

Healthcare teams often lack a systems focus; people tend to work within their own silos. Healthcare workers try to optimize patient care and patient flow within these microsystems, but they often understand little of what goes on in other parts of the hospital. You need a leader who can bridge these gaps, and such leadership comes from a high-level officer.

A MODEL FOR SYSTEM LEADERSHIP

- The executive leadership group designates a senior-level person to provide overall guidance to the team

- A system leader is someone with enough clout in the organization to institute change, with the authority to allocate the time and resources necessary to achieve the team's aim

- It is important that this person have authority over all areas that are affected by the change

- Examples of an appropriate system leader include a vice president for patient services or the director of critical-care medicine

---

Commitment involves a strong will to execute. (We define *will* in this context as the desire to make a difference.) The high Cs need to feel confident that improving performance of the ED will make operations more effective, will boost patient and staff satisfaction and safety, and will have a positive impact on how their hospital is perceived. Resistance within the ranks—which is going to come—will be easier to surmount with the support of administration.

What Is Leadership?

No one's going to argue against the idea that leadership is a good thing to have when you implement a project. But what exactly is leadership—specifically in regard to improving performance in the ED? It is guiding people away from their

---

comfort zone to new systems and processes that not only enhance and improve the patient's experience, but improve the working environment as well.

People fear the unknown. They are comfortable with their current processes. At the most basic level, people are worried about their performance and their jobs rather than anticipating problems in the ED or thinking about ways to improve performance throughout the department or the entire system. For these reasons, many people do not initially embrace change. And many managers struggle to lead change from the status quo.

It is much easier to criticize an effort to improve or change than it is to lead or participate.

One of the primary challenges in improving performance is overcoming this inertia. People within a system commonly think, "If it's not broken, we don't need to fix it." They react to change by keeping their heads down and hoping that this too shall pass. It is difficult for people to envision a system that is different from what they have now.

It is leaders' responsibility to overcome this inertia and mitigate the natural tendency to oppose change.

Authority and influence

Our goals often exceed our authority. We define *authority* as power or rights delegated or given or an organizational privilege extended. With authority comes responsibility. Every increase in authority is accompanied by an increase in responsibilities, and those responsibilities often exceed that authority. (Therefore, it is far better to seek authority than responsibility!) Clearly, having top leaders involved in an ED overhaul brings necessary authority to the project. But many other leaders and participants in the project will still lack the authority required to achieve the goals.

Authority involves power. We define *power* as the ability to influence events and outcomes in your favor. Clearly, power involves more than simply authority. It includes the notion of influence, which is the key to leading beyond a given level of authority. We define *influence* as the capacity to produce effects on others by intangible or indirect means.

If you are skeptical that power can be exercised without authority, consider the examp........................enturies of British rule in India, ... a dhoti and a shawl. He was no.....................ed millions of people, and in 1947, n.....................ce. He also helped end two wars be.....................r strikes. We often equate power t.....................ce could be more effective than sin.....................it to do. "An eye for an eye," he.....................rld is blind."

This con.....................t element of leadership.

Acting as a leader

Perhaps the best way to answer the question "What is leadership?" is to consider what leaders should do—and what they should not do. For example, leaders should:

- Coach and mentor

- Push through barriers

- Establish stretch goals

- Stay in touch with improvement efforts

- Monitor, support, and sustain accountability for progress toward achieving goals

- Commit the necessary resources (time, staff, and money)

- Analyze metrics and ensure that goals are met

Fear of change is the main roadblock to improving the ED. Leaders must replace anxiety with urgency. To overcome anxiety, fear, anger, and resistance, the best method is to communicate, communicate, communicate. You cannot over communicate. And you should use multiple communication channels.

One action required of a leader may seem obvious—so obvious that it may slip by unnoticed (and perhaps unacted on): Leaders must understand the need for change before anything else happens (says John Kotter in *Leading Change*, 1996). They should also identify the change required. In the first chapter, we referred to Don

Berwick's point that any system is designed to produce the results it does. So one of the first steps a leader should take is to examine how the system works and then determine what processes and practices encourage the results the system produces and therefore need to be changed.

Once a leader has identified what needs changing and what sort of change is required (always keeping in mind the prerequisite of involving top leadership), then that leader is responsible to lead the ED and the system through that change. Kotter described the following eight principles for leading change:

1. Establish a sense of urgency

2. Form a powerful guiding coalition

3. Create a vision

4. Communicate the vision

5. Empower others to act on the vision

6. Plan for and create short-term wins

7. Consolidate improvements and produce more change

8. Institutionalize new approaches

Two ways of looking at change may help leaders understand guiding an ED through it. One is that change is a process, not an event. Optimizing the ED means improving performance over time. This effort will not take several months or quarters. It will take nine to 12 months (and maybe one to two years) to boost both performance and satisfaction to the levels you want them to reach. The second is that you are not just changing structures and processes, you are transforming a culture. Embarking on cultural change is one of the most complex tasks you can undertake; it requires patience, humor, and tenacity. This notion that you are transforming a culture helps explain why people can resist change so strenuously.

Change is an art; resistance is a science.

Followers want comfort and stability, but they also want solutions. During this process, you will need to ask hard questions, ones that will knock people out of their comfort zones, and the result will be distress, which you will need to manage. You will encounter a lot of "No"s, so you must be optimistic and encouraging. However, do not ignore or criticize vocal resisters early on; instead, get them on board. Once converted, they can be the best advocates for the process of improvement, or as we call them, "sponsors." Getting them on board involves creating a vision, communicating it, and empowering others.

A leader takes people where they want to go. A great leader takes people where they don't necessarily want to go, but ought to be.
—Rosalynn Carter

Changing a culture may seem like a daunting task, but once transformed, benefits flow naturally from the change. Jim Collins, in his book *Good to Great* (2001), lists principles of what he terms level-five leaders. One involves creating a culture of discipline. When you have people who are disciplined, he notes, you don't need hierarchy. When you have thought that is disciplined, you don't need bureaucracy. When you have action that is disciplined, you don't need excessive controls. In other words, if you empower others who buy into your vision, they'll carry your process of change along.

What's in it for me?

A program for top-level ED performance cannot simply be installed. Management cannot just mandate improvement. It requires the active participation of key ED leaders, as well as other staff. Our goal is commitment, not just compliance.

Level-five leaders, Collins argues, are more like Socrates than Caesar. They have a paradoxical combination: personal humility and professional will. Don't mistake them—they are highly ambitious, but their ambition is first and foremost for the institution, not themselves. Their authority grows out of their influence.

A useful principle to keep in mind throughout the process of improvement is:

Never expect anyone to engage in behavior that serves your values unless you give them a reason to do so.

Ultimately, of course, keeping the patient as the central focus of everything in the process allows us to attain quality, safety, and service. But we also need to consider the needs and desires of the staff. For them, you always need to answer the question "What's in it for me?" Emphasizing enlightened self-interest is one of the keys to involving people in your efforts to transform the culture. Thus, you continually need to keep the following two questions in mind:

- Is this good for the patient?

- Is this good for the healthcare team?

One of the benefits of improving flow in the ED, and one of the goals of a project to improve flow, is making the department a better place to work and the work more satisfying. Other benefits and goals of improved flow are patient satisfaction, patient safety, and improved financial performance. Achieving these goals makes life better for the people on your team. Emphasizing this point and these benefits should be an important part of creating and sharing your vision.

Empowering the staff extends beyond sharing a vision that includes self-interest. Involving two groups—physicians and nurses—in all phases of your improvement project is crucial. The Institute for Healthcare Improvement makes this point: "Engage the physicians in the quality work of the organization; engage [the] organization in the quality work of physicians."[2] Physicians are usually not early adopters of change. They have been trained to be independent, and they have also been highly acculturated, so they likely do not see themselves as part of the problem. When we on-board a new facility, we spend a significant part of our time interacting with physicians, earning their trust, and then getting agreement on vision, mission, values, and goals for the department as well as for their practice. Leaders are not likely to improve a system without the enthusiasm, knowledge, cultural clout, and personal leadership of physicians. Obtaining nursing buy-in is also critical. These two groups may not agree on the mission, so empowering them and helping them see your vision is an important foundation for your improvement project's success.

Let's talk

Systems with a strong patient service culture have several characteristics:

- Team members share a commitment to common goals

- The espoused values are the system's real values

- The team speaks a common language

- A spirit of teamwork and accountability pervades the system, with a sense of looking out for each other and for the goals of the team

One way to achieve this atmosphere is dialogue. Leaders should create a dialogue for problem solving that includes identification of problems, proposal of options and solutions, planning, and support. Effective dialogue is essential to helping your subordinates or team members solve problems and move forward. Use open-ended questions to create dialogue and accomplish mutual goals for you and your organization. Talk with doctors, nurses, and others, using such questions as:

- What do you think about this idea?

- What do you think is important?

- How would you solve this?

- If you were in my shoes, what would you do?

- What other factors should we be considering?

- In your opinion, why is this approach going to work?

- What do you see as the obstacles we face?

Whether you are working with your team as a group or one-on-one, open-ended questions require respondents to share their thinking and enable them to propose ideas. Problem-solving questions should flow from the global to the specific. Figure 2.1 shows types of questions you might ask in various categories.

FIGURE 2.1

OPEN-ENDED QUESTIONS

Global:

- How are things going?

- What are your goals?

- What are you trying to accomplish?

Problem identification:

- What results have you achieved so far?

- Where are you stuck?

- What kinds of problems are you encountering?

     The Hospital Executive's Guide to Emergency Department Management

FIGURE 2.1

OPEN-ENDED QUESTIONS (CONT.)

Options and solutions:

- What solutions have you attempted?

- What do you see as your options?

- Do you want input from me?

Planning:

- What is your "go forward" plan?

- How can you apply what you've learned to your job?

- Who else would benefit from knowing this?

Support:

- What can I do to better support you?

- Whose support do you need?

- Would it be helpful to talk again?

Adapted from Thomas Crane, The Heart of Coaching.[3]

Display your commitment

Making visible the commitment from top leaders helps create this atmosphere of teamwork. Leaders should get out on the "shop floor"—go into the ED when it is busy and follow the path that a patient would take. Look at the waiting room. Is it clean? Is it friendly? Is it conducive to good patient care? Are patients being acknowledged as they arrive? How is the greeter or service person behaving? Is he or she keeping patients and families informed? How are people being treated? What are they doing while they wait? What is it like to walk around to the back of the department? The ED team may be busy, but do they seem concerned about patients and are they treating them with concern and respect? Talk to some of the patients while they are waiting to be treated and after they have been treated to get a sense of what their experiences were like.

Leaders should also talk to the physicians and nursing staff members. Do they feel fulfilled in their work, with a sense that they are accomplishing their mission? Repeat this process on all your units and floors, both when things are quiet and when things are busy. Making yourself available and making your commitment to positive change visible demonstrates your commitment to and passion for improving the experience for your patients and your people.

It's just political

How often have you heard someone say, in a disapproving tone, "It's just politics" or "It was a political decision"? But what is politics? Here's our definition: Politics is about solving problems with competing agendas and scarce resources. An example from the ED is if you have both ED boarders and catheterization patients, who gets upstairs first? Politics in this sense—solving problems—is important to keep in mind when making a process of improvement work, particularly in the early stages. Achieving results means practicing politics, specifically actions such as:

- Building relationships

- Making friends

- Seeking allies

- Creating networks

- Avoiding making enemies

- Rewarding loyalty and integrity

- Being consistent

Your goal should be to maintain relationships and get results at the same time. Always see people as potential resources, not competitors for resources, and treat them that way. Maintaining and developing relationships is an important component of getting people on your team to share your vision and showing them how the changes are also in their interest. Effective persuasion is a learning and negotiation process for leading your colleagues to a shared solution to a problem. Persuasion is not begging or cajoling, selling or convincing; it's learning and negotiating. President Lyndon B. Johnson described politics graphically and bluntly:

It's better to have your enemies inside the tent
pissing out than outside the tent pissing in.

Political issues will arise as you proceed, because there are competing agendas for time, energy, and resources. Initial resisters can become sponsors of your agenda, but don't forget the innovators, early adopters, and people who are on board from the start. Take advantage of their presence and work with them. Identify the sources of power and influence, allies, and change agents early in the process.

Keep the whole process as transparent as possible. And of course, communicate, communicate, communicate.

Inevitably, you will encounter resistance that you can't convert into support. You can't please everybody. Some people will be hurt or adversely affected by the change. Never underestimate the power of a person to protect his or her rice bowl. Sometimes, you will have to transfer the hardcore resisters or otherwise part ways.

Political issues will also arise when there is a misalignment of the mission of the ED. For example, some of the staff members believe they are there just to take care of the very sick, whereas others think they are there to see every patient in a timely fashion. And many staff members may fall somewhere in between these poles. There are different incentives between the physicians, nurses, and staff members in the ancillary services. There are likely differing views on the results of improving flow, as well. Having more patients means what to whom? Getting these issues into the open and reaching an agreement is essential for the ED to carry out its mission. If you do not resolve these conflicts, they can interfere with achieving defined goals for throughput and patient flow. The resulting discord can also take a great deal of effort to manage and resolve.

What Leadership Isn't

Management is about coping with complexity; leadership is about coping with change, notes Kotter. In the long run, both management skills and leadership skills are essential to engage the team, to engage the healthcare system, and to be successful. But they are different sets of skills. Managers look within the current operation to achieve results by:

- Organizing staff members and monitoring performance

- Planning, budgeting, and allocating resources

- Delivering predictable results

- Controlling, reviewing, and solving problems

By contrast, leaders look outside the current boundaries to determine future success by:

- Establishing direction, goals, and standards

- Aligning people and resources with goals

- Motivating and inspiring people

- Measuring progress and making strategic choices

- Producing useful change

- Making patients happy, rewarding employees, and satisfying shareowners

Managers are essential to the long-term success of an operation. But leaders are who people will follow into a battle.

It is also important to know what actions leaders should not take or what qualities they should not have. Someone who is not an effective leader:

- Does not earn trust

- Behaves inconsistently with reality

- Exhibits short-term thinking

- Is unethical

- Cannot articulate a vision with a strategy

- Resists change

- Focuses on self rather than the organization

- Does not find balance in work, family, and self

The Effective Healthcare Improvement Leader

The most important action a leader needs to take is to create trust so that others are inspired to follow where the leader is going. Many of the qualities of a strong leader are the same qualities that make a decent human being—consider the qualities that are the reverse of the negative attributes just listed. A couple of other qualities that fit that description and are vital in leading a project to optimize an ED are a thirst for continuous learning and improvement and a recognition that failure will occur and we need to learn from it. Business virtues that are important include awareness that people are the most important assets of a business and recognition that customers (patients) are why the business (practice) exists. (See Figure 2.2 for the roles the senior leaders of ED improvement projects should fill.)

FIGURE 2.2
A MODEL FOR EXECUTIVE LEADERSHIP

Senior leaders play the following three important roles:

- Sponsor the team

- Create the vision of the new system

- Foster necessary cooperation throughout the system to achieve the organization's goals

To successfully fulfill these roles, senior leaders should:

- Provide overall guidance to the ED team

- Ensure communication by and involvement of senior leadership in the progress of the work

- Ensure that the aims of the change process align with the organization's strategic goals

---

This change is brought to you by ...

You've analyzed why change is necessary and what changes should happen to improve the performance of your ED. You've brought top leadership in your system on board. But when you begin to implement your process of change, you're going to need allies. Now is the time to find sponsors. Any staff members enthusiastic about the process you're about to introduce will be useful and will be valuable allies. They help drive the improvement efforts. They are necessary. However, sponsorship entails some specific attributes, and they involve character-istics of leadership.

ATTRIBUTES OF A SPONSOR

- Basic knowledge of the improvement project

- Authority to muster resources and remove system barriers in the organization

- Direct connection to senior leadership

- Understanding that his or her responsibilities include the success of the improve-ment team

- Alignment of administrative position and responsibilities with the improvement team

---

Sponsors work closely with leadership to connect the improvement project to organizational priorities, help build the will to improve throughout the depart-ment and the system, attain agreement on the aim of the team's work, and develop a strategy to spread the work of the team.

Typically, sponsors help select team members and help the team secure the resources it needs (especially support from the information technology, HR, finance, and similar departments). They keep track of the team's progress, influ-ence its tempo, and monitor how the team's work affects the rest of the system.

They also help communicate progress to the management team. The following are some strategies that help make a sponsor effective:

- Tell inspiring stories across the organization to make the improvement truly align with organizational strategy

- Start small and work up to the full role of sponsor

- Sometimes just observe and keep quiet at team meetings and then follow up with the team leader

- Hold clinicians more accountable and keep them engaged in the improvement effort

Developing leaders

Developing leaders is a long-term process. You begin with recruiting and hiring, but you should continue providing support, including coaching. Another aspect of developing leaders is empowerment. By involving staff members in developing leaders, you empower many people on your staff, and the growth of leaders flows naturally from this process. This growth will even affect recruiting and hiring, which may seem unrelated. The ED is the front door to the hospital, and we view emergency physicians and midlevel providers as "front-door ambassadors" for your hospital and its medical staff, so hiring carefully and providing full support to those individuals is essential. Another of Collins' principles in *Good to Great* is "first who, then what." Any process of improvement begins with getting the right people on the team, the wrong people off the team, and the right people in the right positions. Only then can you move to considering process changes.

Trust me

Lack of strong leadership is a serious deficiency in an ED, often resulting in deteriorating service in multiple areas over several years. Ensuring provision of able leadership by the ED medical director is crucial. In our experience, most medical directors are mature individuals unused to being in a student-mentor position. Gaining the trust of the medical director through a healthy and open relationship and providing transparent goals and metrics is imperative to gradually developing a mentoring process. You should assess—in a subtle but honest and accurate way—the director's skills, strengths, and weaknesses. The medical director will often be open to coaching, as long as it occurs in a professional, collaborative manner. Collaborative mentoring allows you to improve deficiencies and reinforce what is already working well.

Keep in mind as you mentor the medical director and other staff members that "positive reinforcement does not judge people on their past performance, but on their present behavior," according to Aubrey Daniels in *Other People's Habits*.[4] You're going into the future, not into the past. Part of developing leadership is giving people the opportunity to grow. (See how to assess the medical director's strengths and weaknesses and review a sample tool assessment in Figures 2.3 and 2.4.)

FIGURE 2.3

BESTPRACTICES ED DIRECTOR OPERATIONAL SKILLS ASSESSMENT TOOL™

Proficiency	How I rate my skill level (scale of 1 to 5)	Important for me to improve now? (scale of 1 to 5)
ED management		
• Recruiting		
• Staffing and retention		
• Scheduling		
Managing professionals—evaluating, teaching, coaching, and mentoring		
Nursing operations		
Customer service/patient satisfaction—a model and a change package		
Risk management and risk reduction		
Billing and coding		
Performance improvement—rapid-cycle testing and implementation		
ED operations and patient flow		
• Forecasting patient flow		
• Demand capacity management		
• Queuing theory		
Organizational dynamics		
Change management		
Leadership theories and management		
Theory of Constraints		

Rating scale: 1 = Strongly agree   2 = Agree   3 = Neither agree nor disagree   4 = Disagree
5 = Strongly disagree

FIGURE 2.4

PERSONAL LEADERSHIP QUALITIES OF A BESTPRACTICES MEDICAL DIRECTOR™

Qualities	
Courteous and professional	
Enthusiastic	
Willing to go the extra mile	
Encourages teamwork, team player	
Has a commitment to service, safety, and quality	
Good listener	
Synthesizes the opinions of others	
Good project manager	
Has a sense of humor	
Self-aware—doesn't take him- or herself too seriously	
Effective and punctual in meetings	
Manages with integrity	
Familiar with key department metrics and drivers	
In decision-making, errs on the side of service, safety, and quality	
Can articulate the BestPractices balanced scorecard goals and related performance improvement plans and projects	
Integrates ED performance improvement plans into the hospital's strategic and tactical plans	

       The Hospital Executive's Guide to Emergency Department Management

Developing a Shared Governance Model

An effective way to empower others and to develop leaders is to create an ED leadership council. Such a group consists of a cross-section of the ED staff, both permanent members by virtue of position and representative members from various groups. The permanent members include the medical director and nursing director, as well as charge nurses or assistant managers for each shift. When one of these persons is replaced on staff, the newcomer takes on the role of a permanent member; the task should be written into the job description as a function of the position. The representative members of the council should come from staff groups across the ED: physicians, nurses, technicians, unit clerks, and so on.

The number of representative members can vary, depending on the characteristics of the department. Councils that are too large or too small can be ineffective. A sample of representation is one RN per shift, one technician per shift, one unit clerk per shift (or, for smaller departments, one such position, period). The staff groups as configured by the representation pattern should choose the representatives. In other words, all RNs should choose a member if that person is to represent all RNs; if each shift of RNs has a representative member, then only RNs on that shift choose that member.

The staff needs to understand that as the improvement process unfolds, future decisions are up to them because of this council. Making sure they understand this point is part of sharing the vision and empowering the staff.

Leaders should introduce the notion of the leadership council at a joint staff meeting on the topic (you should already be holding regular joint staff meetings involving all ED staff members, including doctors). Give as much detail as possible about the purpose, need, and rationale for the council. To succeed, you must share everything you know with the staff (within certain strategic limitations). Ensure that the staff buys into how the process will work and what its benefits will be. Allow time for questions, and answer every one before moving ahead. Solicit recommendations for representatives and give a clear deadline for submissions.

This is one case that should not be political. You don't want the process to start as a political event or popularity contest. A deadline within a short time from the end of the meeting will decrease the chances of it becoming politicized. You will be surprised: De facto or informal leaders will emerge, and you will have already experienced your first benefit of the council the staff chose. Had you chosen the very same people, the staff's vested interest in success would not be the same.

As soon as the staff chooses its representative members, announce the council and congratulate those recommended. The medical director and nursing director should meet individually with the new council members to ensure their willingness to serve and go over the requirements for doing so. Schedule your first meeting with enough notice to ensure that all team members can participate without scheduling conflicts.

Create the agenda for the first meeting. The following is a sample:

- Welcome members

- Clearly define and explain their roles

- Create and adopt the council's mission statement

- Develop guiding principles

- Schedule set meeting dates

- Define standing agenda headings

Ensure that each member understands his or her role. The mission statement should address these questions: What are we trying to accomplish by forming this council? What are our guiding principles? For example, "We will always strive to practice evidence-based medicine and nursing." The scheduled meeting dates should be regular: the third Tuesday of every month, for example. Creating a regular schedule helps ensure that all team members will be available for meetings.

The standing agenda headings are categories that will help ensure follow-through and success. Agenda items should always fall into one of these headings. Subsections under each heading of new business and old business will facilitate follow-through. The headings are:

- Operations

- Quality

- Safety

- Customer service

- Financial

The role of ED leadership

ED leaders prepare the agenda for each meeting, including presenting new items. These should include opportunities for improvement and problems, as well as possible solutions and solicitation of others. The primary role of the leader is that of facilitator; accordingly, the leader votes only in the case of a tie. (You should create a council with an even number of voters so that if there is a tie, you make the decision.) Explain at the initial meeting that ED leadership can veto actions if necessary, but that the medical director and nursing director must agree on a veto.

The role of the council

As you proceed with plans to improve the operations of your ED, the ED leadership council is going to make decisions in all facets of the project, such as:

- Operational changes and testing

- Hiring

- Staff scheduling

- Quality concerns and initiatives

- Safety concerns and initiatives

- Peer review for clinical concerns

- Service standards and accountability

Benefits to ED leadership and the department

Forming a leadership council, allowing the staff to choose council members, and then giving the council authority to make decisions empowers the people on your staff. They become involved in the project and motivated to succeed. Looking at the broad range of activities under the council's purview gives you an idea of the kind of benefits this model can provide. For example, hiring decisions often involve an element of luck. When leaders hire, they often rely on instincts. However, bringing the council into the process gives you multiple perspectives from concerned parties. Making the staff members part of the process gives them a vested interest in the success of new employees. This involvement and these multiple perspectives give you a better chance of successful hiring. Therefore, present the candidates to the council and let it choose.

Take operations, for example. A council examining every facet of service operations develops council members who continuously search for ways to improve once they are part of a few successes. They also explain and defend decisions to coworkers, describing the process used to tackle the dilemma and explaining why decisions were made. Staff members can usually live with decisions as long as they understand how and why these decisions came about.

The natural leaders who emerge will develop skills and experience that will pay off as your improvement process continues and when you reach the point of maintaining a successful program. Ultimately, this benefit may be the most significant. Creating the next generation of leaders should always be our priority, to leave our organizations better off because we were there.

Carrying Through: A Seminar Is Never Enough

Our organization has a superb patient satisfaction course that energizes most participating clinicians and staff members. The result is a considerable enthusiasm for customer service that lasts for two to four or perhaps four to eight weeks and then dies down. The challenge is embedding new behaviors into the operation. Getting the early adopters to assume new skills and habits is easy. Changing behavior in the majority is more difficult. Research on behavioral change[5] confirms this tendency: 40% of participants will change after a seminar. After an interactive learning experience with follow-up coaching, change increases dramatically. We have built this pattern into our process.

Following the process of empowering staff members, leading them through transforming the culture, and developing leaders as you go into the future will go a long way toward embedding new behaviors into your operation. Remember the four key principles for facilitating change, which are:

1. Make it easy to say "yes"

2. Plan for the conditions that are necessary

3. Build in incentives

4. Ensure commitment from the top

References

1. Kotter, J. *Leading Change*. Boston: Harvard Business School Press, 1996.

2. Reinertsen, J.L., Gosfield, A.G., Rupp, W., Whittington, J.W. "Engaging Physicians in a Shared Quality Agenda". IHI Innovation Series white paper. Cambridge, Massachusetts: Institute for Healthcare Improvement; 2007.

3. Crane, T. *The Heart of Coaching: How to Use Transformational Coaching to Create a High-Performance Coaching Culture*. Third edition. San Diego: FTA Press 2005.

4. Daniels, A., *Other People's Habits*. New York: McGraw-Hill, 2001.

5. Prochasska, J., Norcross, J., Diclemente, C. In Search of How People Change, *American Psychologist*, Sept. 1992.

Fielding Your Best Team

In the 2010 Winter Olympics, the Canadian hockey team was full of National Hockey League stars—and not just stars, but many of the best players in the league. As the Olympic hockey tournament got under way, NHL coach Paul Maurice observed that the Canadians "have the most talented group, the most elite players" in the Olympics. "They have so many talented players," he went on, "that in stretches it's like they're just playing a talent game. … When Canada gets to the point where the talent is secondary and they're playing a team style, that's when they're going to be really tough to beat."[1] Contrast this with the 2010 French National Soccer Team. Considered one of the top teams in the world going into the 2010 World Cup, their subsequent exit was dubbed "Le Meltdown" by the press. After one player was expelled for cursing at the coach, the rest of the team refused to practice, shunned their fans and ultimately lost to South Africa, going home in disgrace.

If you've followed sports for any length of time—any team sport—you've probably witnessed a good team defeat a more talented team simply because they worked together better as a team. This same lesson can be applied to emergency medicine. To be the best ED you can be, you want to have your best team working at all times, and you want your ED staff to work as a high-performance team, not just a collection of skilled providers.

> **Team:** Two or more people who achieve a mutual goal through interdependent actions—not a group that achieves its goal through independent, individual contributions. The essential elements of a team include a common purpose and shared goals, interdependent actions, communication, accountability, and a collective effort.

Hire Right: A Team Vs. B Team

Hiring right is critical, but it does not mean hiring only the most skilled individuals or the persons with the strongest resumes. You need to look at some important attributes of the individuals you consider, including qualities that influence how well they'll fit into your team. A concept we've often used is A Team versus B Team. You want to avoid hiring B Team members.

The surest route to having the kind of ED you want is hiring and keeping the right people. You want A Team members.

A Team members do things the right way. They come to work early and with energy. They are committed to working with the team. An approach we've found useful when you're hiring and as you're developing leadership is to diagram contrasting attributes of A Team and B Team members:

A Team characteristic:	B Team characteristic:
Positive	Negative
Proactive	Reactive
Confident	Poor communicator
Competent	Late
Compassionate	Lazy
Team player	Constant complainer

Finding the A Team

How do you get the best team of professionals into your ED? Undoubtedly, you have from time to time hired a B Team person and been a member of the "hire in haste, repent at leisure" club. Thinking about teamwork characteristics when hiring emphasizes the benefit of involving the leadership council in the process. Doing so offers a complete assessment of candidates' teamwork qualities from people who will be working with them on your team. Keeping such attributes in mind also underscores the importance of checking multiple references and asking questions to gauge to what extent the candidates likely possess these qualities.

Another way of approaching the task is to look at your department first before even thinking about the candidates. Ask yourself what your department needs. Consider the following questions:

- Does your ED need a major overhaul or does it just need fine-tuning?

- Is your ED functioning within benchmark standards?

- Do you have stable nursing leadership within your ED?

- Is the medical staff supportive of the ED?

- What specialty groups complain the most about the ED? Why do they complain?

- What do your patients tell you about the ED?

- Within your community, what is the preferred ED?

For example, benchmark standards include measures such as staffing ratios, productivity, length of stay, number of patients who've left without being seen, ancillary turnaround times, level of patient satisfaction, etc. Stable nursing leadership is a nurse manager or director who has been in place successfully for more than two years. When considering complaints by specialty groups, ask yourself whether their complaints are legitimate. In regard to patient comments, are patients concerned about wait times, or your providers, or nursing staff?

You need to fully understand the condition your ED is in before you can determine how you would like it to be. Only then can you establish a realistic plan for successfully moving from where you are to where you want to go. Having this sense of where you are and where you need to go will also help you determine what sorts of qualities you're likely to need in candidates to help you succeed in attaining your goal. You should expect a great deal from the physician leadership, and you should carefully assess the characteristics of the persons on your team, including their abilities to engage in effective teamwork, before you place anyone in a leadership role.

A Critical Step: Hiring the Medical Director

Gaining clarity on the current state of your department and determining where you want it to be provides a valuable foundation as you set out to hire the medical director. When you begin the process of hiring the right person for that position, remember that your team should be involved in recruiting and interviewing candidates. The team members involved in the process should agree on key attributes necessary for an effective medical director for your ED. You should coordinate the interviewing and ensure that interviewers have a structure to help them evaluate the candidate's potential to succeed. The interviewing team should also explain in writing your expectations of the director and the challenges that person will face and review them with each candidate.

Skills expected of medical directors

We use a standard contract in employing medical directors that spells out such expectations in detail. We focus on the following nine characteristics.

Communication: being accessible

The medical director should be available by telephone, voice mail, pager, or e-mail. When unavailable, the director must ensure that the department can contact an administrative representative when it needs administrative assistance. The medical director must respond rapidly to pages and to other forms of contact. Quick response is essential in this position. We provide secure communication through intranet and an e-mail address and expect medical directors at our contracted facilities to be proficient in using those means and to ensure that all providers at their sites are using them. These tools provide time-efficient ways to communicate in the ED.

Scheduling: being organized

The medical director should be well organized and must establish and then maintain a clearly defined schedule, including shifts and required meetings. Careful ordering of shifts should avoid schedule conflicts—and that ability is imperative in a medical director, as the director's responsibilities include scheduling his or her own clinical shifts. Identifying how the medical director represents the ED to the hospital is important, so creating monthly and weekly schedules that allow the director to complete clinical and administrative responsibilities should be a priority of getting organized. If there are specific days the medical director needs to be in committee meetings or available for administrative responsibilities, they must be noted in advance and arrangements made so the director can be available to fulfill those responsibilities.

In addition, the director typically attends meetings such as the hospital's medical staff committees, the medical executive committee, medicine and surgery committees (if the ED committee reports to them), emergency medicine committee, monthly site medical director conference calls, and semiannual leadership conferences. The director should participate in pediatrics, cardiovascular surgery, OB/GYN, and other hospital committees whenever they require contributions from the ED. However, note that the director shares responsibilities for attending these meetings with the assistant medical director.

Group meetings of this sort may seem routine or even a chore, but they are essential for ensuring clear communication with the physician group. Meetings solely for providers may take place after hospital meetings. Topics that should be the

    The Hospital Executive's Guide to Emergency Department Management

focus of meetings at least every two months are continuous quality improvement, chart review, medical staff issues, department flow issues, and similar subjects.

Reporting: maintaining accurate and timely records

Some of the responsibilities we outlined earlier in the chapter no doubt seem unexciting. Maintaining accurate and timely records is one. But these unexciting tasks are vital in your effort to attain high quality. They should not be overlooked or have their importance underestimated. They affect both smooth flow and clear communication. The director (or his or her administrative assistant) maintains records regarding meeting attendance, department issues, facility issues, and continuing quality improvement, and he or she should review the results with the chief medical officer quarterly. These records also come under review in the monthly conference calls of medical directors to ensure clear companywide communication.

Ensuring quality: maintaining and improving metrics

Clearly, maintaining quality as you proceed in your project and improving it is essential to your ED's success. You can track the quality of your department's work either on paper or electronically using a computer program. The medical director should ensure that tracking occurs and metrics are reviewed regularly. When addressing quality, organizations should focus on several points, such as:

- Patient complaints

- X-ray overreads and positive culture result logs

- Standard chart audits

- Key Centers for Medicare & Medicaid Services (CMS) requirements, such as medication administration times for myocardial infarction and community-acquired pneumonia

The high-quality ED deals with patient complaints rapidly and resolves them. The director should ensure that information on complaint management is readily available to hospital administration and provides enough detail to clearly convey how the department is handling complaints. We cannot overemphasize how important good customer service is in the ED, just as it is in any other business.

X-ray overreads and positive culture result logs are vital to ensure quality and desirable patient outcomes. The director should hold each physician accountable for ensuring that any discrepancies are handled accurately and quickly. If the medical director does not ensure this compliance, these activities will often fall through the cracks, and mismanagement of the patient will occur. Such mismanagement carries potentially serious medical and legal implications.

Standard chart audits include a 72-hour return evaluation. Charts of patients who have a 72-hour return admission should be audited. You may forward the printout for 72-hour returns to the medical records department, and you should closely review all 72-hour return admits every month for problems and lessons learned.

The director should also ensure that the ED closely tracks all of CMS' core quality measures. This means the director will need to work closely with the data extractor to ensure that the department obtains the correct information in a timely fashion so that the organization can attain these goals. These are high-priority goals.

Accomplishing them is critical. For example, the medical director should monitor the percentage of patients with transient neurological symptoms and intermittently audit charts for diagnosis and length of stay. Carry out trauma audits with the trauma coordinator.

When a physician does not interact with patients or provide clinical care with the quality or consistency expected, the medical director should work with that physician on quality improvement. The director can suggest that the physician enroll in continuing medical education or other outside education courses. The director can also provide coaching in counseling sessions. The director should document these sessions. For midlevel providers, such as nurse practitioners and physician assistants, we suggest auditing about 5% of their patient visits. The midlevel manager or lead staff member should conduct initial reviews and forward them to the director, who should review any problem charts thoroughly. The midlevel manager then should educate and counsel the providers, working with the medical director when concerns about clinical competency arise. All such actions to improve quality are confidential. However, they should be documented and maintained in the staff member's file, clearly marked to indicate continuous quality improvement.

Administering: communication again

Administration often implies routine, necessary (but unexciting) activities that may seem unrelated to your improvement project. Understanding where these fit into the improvement equation requires understanding that administration is all about communication. Specifically, it calls for the medical director to arrange monthly or bimonthly meetings with the hospital CEO and the key administrator (chief medical officer, vice president of medical associates, or the equivalent) overseeing operations in the ED. This regular channel of communication enables you to head off potential problems, maintain high quality once it's attained, and stay on track. Similarly, the director should keep open communication ongoing with the hospital's chief of staff or chief medical officer and should review any medical staff issues and help resolve them quickly.

Routine activities still require clear procedures and documentation. For example, for department expenses, our contract clearly states that the administrative assistant should coordinate the purchase of office supplies, and the monthly expense report should include all other expenses, those for recruiting as well as maintenance of the ED.

Monitoring staffing

Another facet of the medical director's role is forming and maintaining the schedule. Ultimately, the buck stops here: The director is responsible for making sure that the ED has the necessary physicians and staff to cover each shift. Doing so may involve rapid, direct communication with the physicians within the medical group. It may also mean the director fills a position to avoid lapses in coverage. The midlevel manager should determine hours of coverage by midlevel providers, consulting with the director as necessary.

If your hospital contracts with emergency service providers, you should define performance expectations and define coverage and staffing parameters to the extent that you understand them. Whether you contract with an outside group or employ your own ED physicians, you can use this approximate rule of thumb: You can satisfactorily cover your ED professional staffing needs based on the productivity of the clinical staff, which is often set at two patients per hour. An ED with 50,000 annual visits, in other words, will require 25,000 provider staff hours annually. Generally, emergency physicians will work about 144 hours per month or 1,728 hours per year. Under this formula, your department would require 14.5 full-time equivalents. Midlevel providers can supplement physician staffing. For example, they commonly staff a fast-track unit in the ED because of the reduced acuity and complexity of patients seen there. Some departments use midlevel providers as procedure specialists or practitioners to enhance the efficiency of physicians in the main emergency room.

Recruiting: finding the best team

Leading the staff does not stop at scheduling and monitoring. The director also plays an important role in choosing team members. The director should have responsibility for assessing staffing needs and working with the organization to recruit new physicians. We've emphasized the importance of involving the team in choosing the team, but the leader needs to lead here. The director should take part in all interviews and should review all recruiting files. Although the midlevel manager assumes this role in recruiting midlevel providers, the medical director should take part in these interviews as well. The director should also ensure that once the department hires a physician, the credentialing process progresses smoothly.

Supervising billing

The medical director's role should include ensuring a smooth billing operation. It may seem unglamorous, but this function is critical to becoming a high-quality ED. For example, medical directors should conduct a monthly review of all down-coding information from the agency that handles billing. Once again, clear documentation is vital, so the director should work with physicians to improve performance in documentation. The director should also work with the administrative assistant to ensure smooth chart flow and chart forwarding. If problems arise, the director must resolve them. Additionally, the director and the chief financial officer should review quarterly financial data. (*Note:* We no longer allow professional courtesy because of the Stark Law and the potential for fraud and abuse. Any billing adjustments must be done with great care.)

Reviewing legal issues

The medical director should review any potential malpractice cases, whether they arise from unexpected deaths, misdiagnosis, or any other reason. If a suit is filed, the director should contact the organization's legal counsel immediately and complete appropriate case-tracking forms.

Being the face of the organization

The medical director needs to be visible. Like it or not, the director represents the ED to the hospital and, ultimately, to the public as well. We recognize this role in our contract, which concludes with sections stating that our medical directors represent our organization. "*You* are the 'captain of the ship,' " the contract's final section says. "Rapid response to problems and being available at all times for questions or concerns is essential and required." Ensuring that the ED is a well-functioning unit requires accountability and a "buck stops here" attitude. The director should be approachable, flexible, accessible, and demonstrate A Team behavior.

There is no magic recipe to ensure that you hire a successful team. When choosing a medical director, however, you will increase your potential for success by keeping the following characteristics in mind:

- Successful experience managing EDs

- A positive, can-do attitude

- A commitment to working successfully with nursing staff

- A commitment to understanding the needs of the medical staff while also representing the needs of the department

- A commitment to the community

- An interest and enthusiasm in the growth of the ED and the entire facility

Defining expectations, roles, and responsibilities; creating routine forums for transparent data analysis and clear communication; and insisting on a reasonable balance of administrative time and clinical time are some of the crucial ingredients that heighten the potential for success of a medical director.

The Rest of the Team

Understanding your emergency staffing needs is critical to fielding the right team. So once you've assessed where your ED is now and determined where you want it to go, you're following the right track. To stay on track, start by examining current conditions. Assess your current staff, pay, shifts, and operations economics. Then identify what staffing needs your ED has—how many providers do you need, what type of providers, and what roles will they be filling? Hiring the right medical director is important, but so is the next step: recruiting and hiring the assistant medical director (or identifying one from within the organization). A similar process should follow for employing physicians, midlevel providers, and support staff. In every case, you should interview and check references carefully before you make offers and negotiate contracts (when required). Once you have hired your professional staff members, make sure you credential them as quickly as possible if they are new to the hospital.

Remember as you go through this process to look for persons with A Team characteristics and hire A Team members.

Teamwork Attributes, Tools, and Techniques

Once you've hired your team, other elements come into play. No one wants to be a B Team member. Often in EDs, you hear this type of comment:

> *"It was a good day today because we had good people on."*
> —Shawna J. Perry, MD[2]

Perry raises the question: Are there really bad people who show up for a shift? Do ED staff members come to work with the intent of making it a bad day for everyone? Or is a good day really when a group of staff members are working together effectively as a team? Teamwork behavior and the skills it requires are teachable. Just because someone has superb individual clinical skills does not guarantee he or she will be an effective team player. At the same time, superb teamwork does not replace clinical skills—it augments and enhances them. Teamwork affects every aspect of ED operations: patient safety, patient flow, patient satisfaction, workforce satisfaction, and clinical processes.

Crew resource management and MedTeams

In early 2002, two community hospitals in Rocky Mount, NC, one with 63,000 ED visits per year and the other with 40,000 visits, trained all 18 physicians and 10 physician assistants to use an innovative program that taught teamwork skills. As a result, staff satisfaction and morale increased, patient complaints dropped to zero, and one of the hospitals won a Jackson Group Award for the greatest improvement in patient satisfaction scores over an eight-month period.

The program, called MedTeams, translates a concept developed by the military known as crew-resource management into the medical field. Trained MedTeams not only help decrease human errors but also reduce the number of handoffs and provide easier access to information. They implement systems in which physicians do not have to rely on their memory or vigilance when attending to numerous patients.

When setting up MedTeams or similar programs, the following are five specific objectives you should focus on:

1. Creating an environment conducive to a team structure and teamwork

2. Focusing on a highly trained team: creating the setup for success

3. Planning and problem solving: verbalizing intentions through a system of feedback and checkbacks

4. Managing workload: learning the most effective strategy for working together when multiple traumas are present or the ED is busy

5. Team improvement strategies: implementing coaching, after-event reviews, and formal methods such as grand rounds or patient safety rounds and evaluations

This approach gives you a way to address top performers and low performers in your department. Perry describes the purpose of the MedTeams program as providing "concrete tools for maintaining good communication, improving team performance and quality of care, no matter which staff members are on shift."

Tools of the team

Under this concept, a team in the ED involves virtually any type of staff member: physicians, midlevel practitioners, nurses, technicians, the unit secretary, patient-flow coordinator, and triage personnel. Teamwork skills they learn particularly emphasize verbal behavior. Learning those skills involves some specific practices.

Callouts

The doctor or nurse in charge vocalizes what he or she is doing and what needs to be done: "This patient needs an airway." "Is somebody getting the radiologist?"

Checkbacks

Vocalizing needs can be effective, but orders shouted into thin air are meaningless. If no one responds to a question, the attending physician has no proof that anyone is carrying out the order. Thus, team members voice responses to callouts, and the physician or other member who gave the initial callout confirms the response. The entire ED process runs much more smoothly when staff members use oral callouts and checkbacks.

The two-challenge rule

Team members respectfully challenge the attending physician's orders, not once but twice, if evidence of a potential cognitive error exists. Although cognitive errors occur frequently in EDs, some departments do not support colleagues in voicing challenges. In other departments, if a reply to one challenge does not produce the desired answer, the questioner automatically yields to the attending physician. To decrease errors, a team member must have the right to challenge an order twice. Indeed, staff members are responsible for questioning all actions that could result in harm to the patient. The team member challenged must then explain the action.

Cross-monitoring

The program encourages team members to check in with their teammates when they work with patients and offer assistance. Often in the ED, such a practice would be met with resistance: "You're invading my territory." "You're questioning my competence." Although such reactions may not be voiced, they are thought. The MedTeams method enables colleagues instead to step in and offer help. For example, one can open an airway or attend to a laceration while the other addresses another concern. Studies have confirmed that the quality of care in EDs dramatically improves when colleagues are able to help in this way.

Situational awareness

Situational awareness means knowing what's going on in the department. Communication is essential to achieving it. But the concept extends beyond clear communication. It includes the sense that every individual on the team is responsible for the overall functioning of the ED. No staff person gives up responsibility for what he or she does, but teammates must at all times be aware of how busy the ED is, what other pods are doing, how busy triage is, and so on. Every staff member, in other words, owns a piece of the problem—but also a piece of the solution. One way to encourage situational awareness is holding team meetings at the beginnings of shifts (or during them) to share information about patients.

Challenges to teamwork

When you implement MedTeams or a similar crew resource management program, two challenges involving staff members become apparent. First, with frequent staff turnover, part-timers, and considerable rotation, setting up training times and maintaining consistency can be difficult. Training averages anywhere from six to 24 months, depending on the size and complexity of the ED. Second, staff members often initially resist changing the current culture. However, once you implement such an approach and staff members experience it, resistance often diminishes. In the high-stress, tense environment of emergency medicine, this model allows everyone to contribute and to feel that they belong to the team. Staff satisfaction ranks high among MedTeams since the system not only reduces errors, improves flow, and increases patient satisfaction, but it also makes each team member's job easier and more fun.

As for the training challenge, the Dynamics Research Corporation Institute for Quality Healthcare has developed an orientation for temporary staff members (which could also be used for new staff members before they receive full training) that introduces them to the concept and briefly explains the procedures and the benefits. Here's how it begins:[3]

Welcome to [name of hospital] Emergency Department. At [name of hospital], we take pride in the quality of emergency services we provide to our patients. Essential to the provision of quality services is providing an environment that enables our emergency personnel to be highly successful at what they do. To that end, emergency personnel at [name of hospital] Emergency Department have been trained to function within a structured teamwork system. It is our expectation that all emergency department personnel, including those who are rotators, part-time, or per diem, become familiar with and actively participate in the team system developed by our department. To help with this process we have provided you with this overview. Please take the time to read it completely.

The [Hospital] ED Teamwork System

One of the principles of our teamwork system is a clearly defined team structure. At any given time in our ED there are [number] physicians on duty. There are nursing staff consisting of [name each category of nursing personnel]. In order to recognize which personnel are caring for which patients, we have devised a [type of system—e.g., color-coding] system.

There are typically [number] teams in the ED at any given time: the coordinating team and [number] core teams. Members of the coordinating team include [list members] and are recognized by [identifier]. The role of the coordinating team is to assist the core teams by coordinating resources within the department. Core teams are identified by [identifier]. This process allows you to readily identify members of your own team who can assist you in meeting your patients' needs. The [core team identifiers] are available to staff by [explain process of distribution]. Team assignments are made out by the coordinating team and communicated by [explain process—e.g., listed on the whiteboard]. A physician will be assigned to each team and will assume the role of the team leader.

Just as a smoothly functioning team in sports can win despite not having the most talented players, a smoothly functioning team in the ED can help you attain your goal of a high-quality operation. Teamwork helps reduce errors and improve patient satisfaction. It also leads to smoother flow.

References

1. Alexander, C. *The News and Observer*. The Pressure is on for Team Canada. Feb. 21, 2010.

2. Perry, S. MedTeams: An Approach to Improved Teamwork and Error Reduction. ACEP CQI Newsletter

3. Risser, et al. The Potential for Teamwork. The MedTeams Research Consortium. *Annals of Emergency Medicine*. 1999; 34: 373–383.

Improving Patient Flow

We often hear that the larger the ED, the more time a patient will spend there, and that statement is typically true (see Figure 4.1). Unfortunately, patients do not perceive spending more time in the ED as a good thing. Graphs measuring patient satisfaction show an inverse relation between time spent in the ED and satisfaction.

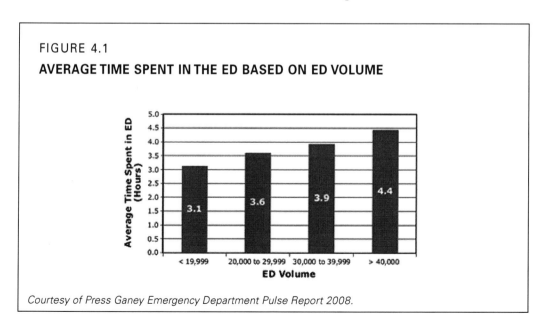

FIGURE 4.1

AVERAGE TIME SPENT IN THE ED BASED ON ED VOLUME

Courtesy of Press Ganey Emergency Department Pulse Report 2008.

You may have a great ED, one with an excellent staff that provides top-notch care, but the more time patients spend with you, the less happy they are. Systems designed without smooth patient flow in mind tend to result in backlogs that produce not only unhappy patients but also dissatisfied staff. Improving flow through the ED leads to more satisfied patients and, in turn, happier staff members who can concentrate on providing excellent care.

Flow is the movement of people and materials through a service system. In healthcare, flow means moving patients through queues and service transitions. Improving flow does not necessarily mean adding space, equipment, and staff members. It means improving the processes in the system. For example, we worked with an ED that averaged 40,000 patient visits per year. We reduced the length of stay by one hour—from three hours to two hours in the main ED and two hours to one hour in the fast-track ED. That reduction of time produced 40,000 new hours of ED capacity. If you divide 40,000 new hours of service capacity by two hours per patient visit, you have the capacity for 20,000 new ED patient visits that you can handle with little to no increase in overhead.

However, improving flow does not mean simply making every process faster. An important principle to keep in mind as you set out to improve flow in the ED is that you want to be fast at fast things and slow at slow things.

For example, a woman in her mid-20s comes to your ED with what clearly appears to be a sprained wrist. Keeping that patient waiting for two hours and then ordering an x-ray is not effective flow. You want to send that patient through the system as quickly as possible. On the other hand, suppose that a man in his late 70s arrives with severe abdominal pain. Taking six hours to examine that patient comprehensively, run tests, and make the proper diagnosis is effective flow. Different types of patients require different journeys through your system and assessing which kind of treatment patients need is an important component of effective patient flow. Your goal is to provide excellent and efficient care in both of the cases we've just described.

The first action you should take to improve flow is to go into the ED and watch what happens. Spend a few hours observing. You'll learn about the processes that are now in place, and you'll also see how what actually occurs diverges from what you thought was supposed to happen. This preliminary work is an important first step.

Next comes the theory. Improving patient flow involves considerable data and analysis. Once you have processes in place to gather data and analyze the results, you're well on your way to improving flow in your department.

Matching Demand with Capacity

If you were to make a graph of the patient arrivals in your department, you'd discover something many others in the United States—who have done this—have learned: There is a predictable pattern. In fact, those many graphs reveal that the pattern is the same everywhere in the country (see Figure 4.2). The number of patients starts to increase around 6 a.m. and goes steadily upward until about 9 a.m., after which it remains level until about 5 p.m., when it starts increasing again, peaking around 10 p.m. After that point, it starts to decline. Knowing this pattern gives us an important piece of information: Patient flow is predictable.

If we know that flow is predictable, then we have the answers to the following two key questions in matching demand with capacity:

1. How many patients are coming?

2. When are they coming?

When we understand this pattern, we can predict with 85% certainty how many patients are coming and when. Being able to predict these patterns helps us address a third key question:

3. Will our service capacity match that demand?

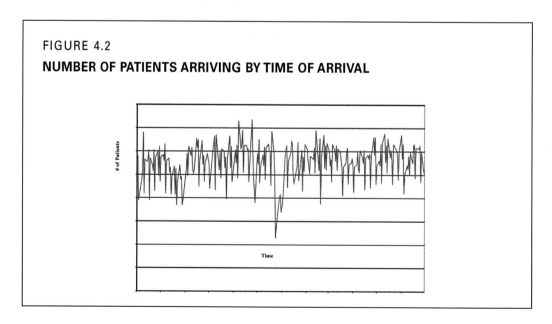

FIGURE 4.2

NUMBER OF PATIENTS ARRIVING BY TIME OF ARRIVAL

    The Hospital Executive's Guide to Emergency Department Management

Most EDs are staffed for averages. Half the time you don't have the resources or staff members you need, and the other half you're overstaffed. In other words, this staffing pattern guarantees that 50% of the time, you are under capacity. If you drew a horizontal line through the curve of Figure 4.2, you'd illustrate how the relationship of demand and capacity in our healthcare system is often handled today.

Even though patient flow is predictable, patient volume is variable. Volume in the slowest and busiest days at smaller EDs often varies by as much as 40%. To configure staffing, you should ask yourself, "What is a reasonable workload for my facility and my physicians?" Today, the complexity and acuity of patient conditions, customer service expectations, skilled workforce shortages, crowding (including boarders), and risk management mean that the number of patients a physician can realistically treat per hour is lower than in the past. A rule of thumb you can use is 1.8 to 2.8 patients per provider per hour. Consider that a year contains 8,760 hours. Look at total volume at different rates of patients per hour (PPH):

- 2 PPH x 8,760 hours/year = 17,520 patients per year

- 2.5 PPH x 8,760 hours/year = 21,900 patients per year

- 3 PPH x 8,760 hours/year = 26,280 patients per year

However, a simple total can be misleading. For example, 18,000 visits during the 8,760 hours in a year equals 2.05 patients per hour, which might seem a reasonable workload for your current staff. But 64% of the daily patient volume in the typical department occurs between 10 a.m. and 10 p.m. So during that time span, the ED that sees 18,000 patients annually on average is treating patients at a rate of 2.63 per hour. Functionally, that volume equals 23,000 visits annually. Thus, it is important to match capacity to demand—at whatever point in the day that demand occurs.

Matching capacity does not automatically mean adding more physicians. In the average ED, physician assistants or nurse practitioners can see up to 30% of arriving patients without a physician's involvement. These midlevel providers are generally more productive in a dedicated fast track than when assisting physicians in the main area.

However, adding staff members is not the only answer to demand–capacity management. Predicting not just how many patients are coming but when they are coming allows you to adjust staffing patterns with existing staff members to better fit the pattern. For example, we worked with one hospital in which the fast track was open from noon to midnight, because the ED seemed to have the heaviest traffic during that time span. But when we analyzed the data, we found that the patients really started coming in around 9 a.m. or 10 a.m. and the ED was still backlogged until midnight to 2 a.m. So we extended the fast-track hours, operating it from 9 a.m. to 1 a.m. As a result, a significantly greater percentage of patients went through the fast track.

Do not overlook the obvious. See when patients are coming and match resources to that time.

Shaping Demand

You can also approach demand–capacity management from the other side by shaping demand. Every winter, we dread flu season because it creates backlogs in the ED. What would happen if you emphasized getting patients—and people in the community—vaccinated for the flu? You may not think of vaccination as part of your ED's mission, but if you vaccinate high-risk patients, you can help shape your winter demand. You can also change your care procedures. For example, start respiratory therapy for arriving asthma patients immediately rather than waiting for the physician. In some cases, giving Solu-Medrol or a dose of PO steroid in triage can reduce the likelihood of admission by 25%–30%. You can encourage walk-in patients to come at nonpeak hours by advertising your slowest hours and offering the prospect of a shorter wait. Alternatively, offer passes (subject to local laws) that give patients priority at another time, similar to Disney's Fast Pass. Patients can choose to wait or come back during a nonpeak time.

To predict demand in your ED, you'll need to evaluate three other principles of flow improvement that are closely linked to demand–capacity management. They are real-time monitoring of patient flow, forecasting, and queuing theory.

Watching, analyzing, and predicting

Driving a car is easier when your dashboard instruments are functioning and visible. Likewise, patient flow in the ED is smoother when you have a functioning dashboard. A simple one might list patients, what labs or tests they're undergoing, and who is treating them. A more complex version, one that is more useful in monitoring patient flow as it's actually happening in an ED, displays multiple screens showing activity in various aspects of ED operations, such as time from arrival of patients to their being seen by a physician or turnaround times for x-rays.

When you monitor cycles as they're occurring, you can see when demand is exceeding capacity; you see exactly what you need, not what you think you might need. You should monitor lab use along with the other aspects of ED operations. As you gather data from your monitoring over time, you can pinpoint when and where backups are forming. For your arriving patients, determine categories based on chief complaint, triage assessments, arrival by emergency medical services, emergency severity index level, and ancillary usage.

All this information, when collated and analyzed, provides valuable insight into the patterns in your ED. This insight will help you forecast future patterns. Use the information you've gathered about demand exceeding capacity when scheduling staffing. Staffing includes not only ED physicians, nurses, and midlevel providers but also lab technicians. If you've assessed patient arrivals with the level of categories suggested previously, you're equipped to answer another key question in demand–capacity management: What will those patients need?

You may think that determining and forecasting patterns is well and good, but what about unusual disruptions of patterns? Patients arriving at an ED represent a system with unscheduled demand. Other examples include a telephone help line or the line at your grocery store. Any system with unscheduled demand will develop a queue at times, a line that forms when more people want the service than the providers can serve at the same time. Queuing theory focuses on how to match fixed resources to unscheduled demand. A theory is possible because engineers have discovered that systems with unscheduled demand follow a set of mathematical principles (Figure 4.3 shows an example from an urgent-care clinic with unscheduled arrivals).

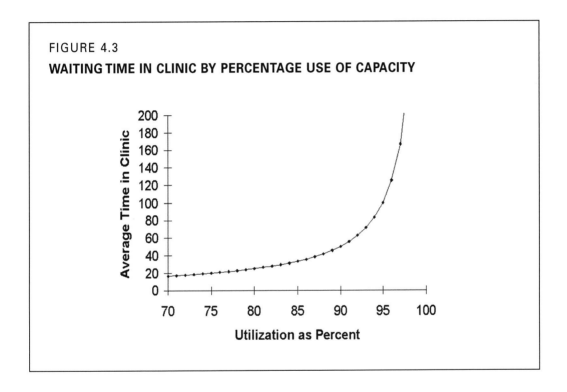

FIGURE 4.3

WAITING TIME IN CLINIC BY PERCENTAGE USE OF CAPACITY

The horizontal axis is utilization as a percentage—is the clinic doctor busy or not busy? The vertical axis is the average time spent in the clinic. As use of the facility increases, the wait time starts to rise. Queuing theory shows, as this graph illustrates, that this curve is not linear; it is logarithmic. It rises gradually to a certain point, and then it really takes off.

Many hospitals' goal is to run at 100% capacity, thinking full capacity is a good thing. The graph shows it is not. If you run at 100% capacity, you guarantee backups and safety issues. People and systems cannot function at 100% capacity and effectively handle variations in volume and complexity. This mathematical equation implies that there is a sweet spot for optimal efficiency when operating a system with unscheduled demand, which is at about 85% of capacity. So if you gear your processes with the goal of operating at 85% of capacity and make use of your forecasting, you'll be in better shape to handle those unexpected spikes in demand.

Constraints and Variations in the System

If we acknowledge that queues are going to form in our system of unscheduled demand, we'll be closer to understanding something significant about healthcare: It is a network of both queues and service transitions. Being a network means that what happens in one part of the network affects other parts of the network and thus the network as a whole. For example, sometimes there are patients who cannot be cared for by midlevel providers, so they are transitioned from triage to emergency physicians. This bogs down staff members when more patient arrive than can be efficiently treated. Queues form and they affect the entire department. The physicians in this case constitute a scare resource. A resource can be a person, a bed, or a piece of equipment. If a resource is likely to become scarce, then it is a constraint.

The Theory of Constraints addresses what happens when resources become scarce, as in our triage example. What happens next is what is known as a bottleneck. Bottlenecks are defined as what happens when the demand for a resource exceeds the capacity of that resource. And because we're in a network, one hour lost at a bottleneck is one hour lost for the whole system.

But not every bottleneck is alike. Systems experience what we call critical and noncritical bottlenecks. This distinction is important operationally. If you improve conditions that create a critical bottleneck, then you improve throughput in the system and you improve flow. However, if you take steps to improve conditions that constitute a noncritical bottleneck, you will not improve overall throughput in the system. Determining what it a critical bottleneck and what isn't can be a challenge, but the main idea is to implement a small change and test it, and then analyze the results. If you find that overall flow has not improved, then the condition you changed is not a critical bottleneck.

Bottlenecks are tricky in another way as well—they can fluctuate. One resource can be a bottleneck at certain times, but at other times, a different resource becomes the bottleneck and the first one ceases to be one. Tracking conditions through real-time monitoring and forecasting them through the collection and analysis of data over time help you determine what is becoming a critical bottleneck (or very likely to become one) at any particular time. If you pinpoint several that occur regularly, fix one and then move on to the next.

Doing what you can do—all the time

If you can keep your resources from becoming constraints in the first place, you'll help keep patients flowing smoothly through the ED. One approach is to ensure that the members of your clinical team perform only the tasks they alone can perform and that they are kept busy in those activities. Be clear on what the role of each position on the team is. Let doctors be doctors and nurses be nurses.

In other words, doctors and nurses should:

- Make diagnostic and treatment decisions

- Manage the team and patient flow

- Function as mobile intellectual resources throughout the ED

- Carry out activities that add value to the process at all times

Similarly, lab technicians should perform only those tasks that they are uniquely qualified to perform.

By contrast, doctors and nurses should not be spending time in activities that are not uniquely their tasks and that anyone could do. A doctor should not be looking for lab tests, entering test requests, or finding x-rays. A nurse should not be doing everything for which no one else has a clearly defined responsibility. In particular, you should guard against having nurses—or physicians—engage in data entry and spend most of their time at a computer terminal.

In his book on the British and American military and political leaders who led the Allies to victory in World War II, Andrew Roberts points out that General Alanbrooke, the British chief of the imperial general staff, concentrated on formulating strategy and advising Winston Churchill on military options. "He was respected in the War Office for being excellent at delegation and almost never got caught up in the details of day-to-day military operations,"[1] Roberts observes, and then comments on this quality:

Like other talented and hard-working individuals at the top of their professions, he only did what only he could do.[2]

Your clinical team members should steadily perform only what they can do. First, keep clinical staff members busy seeing new patients. This concept is crucial to steady flow and to avoid bottlenecks. Focus on getting physicians and patients in a room together as quickly as possible. Physicians are the scarcest resource in the ED, and patient throughput really starts when physicians are together with the patients. To smooth flow, establish processes for ordering simple procedures, such as x-rays, before the doctor sees the patient. In effect, put the physician–patient encounter into triage. Some EDs put a doctor or a midlevel provider in triage to start a workup that someone else takes over at a later stage. This process improves the flow of patients.

Constraints should not have idle time.

If you view physicians as a scarce resource, your goal should be to always have patients for them to see. Structure your ED's processes so that the physicians always have work to do.

The effects of variation

Your ED is full of variation, and that variation affects flow significantly. For example, a Canadian study of 12 physicians found no correlation between diversion and a particular physician—except in regard to two of the physicians. For one physician, patients had a significantly lesser chance of diversion; for the other, patients had a significantly greater chance of diversion. The differences between physicians' styles of treatment are examples of inherent variability—different people deliver services differently. Clinical variability occurs because not every patient suffering from congestive heart failure has the same level of sickness. System variability occurs because patients decide when they want to come to the ED.

Some variation in flow will occur naturally within your system. You predict it, prepare for it, and manage it by using the tools we've discussed—forecasting, monitoring, and matching demand with capacity. The type of variable flow that isn't natural to the system is what we call artificial (e.g., when patients with non-urgent conditions come to the ED). You should try to reduce artificial variation as much as possible to smooth flow.

For example, you can use tools to shape demand. Do more of what already works well. Have you noticed one doctor who keeps patients moving through the system swiftly while still providing excellent care? Does a particular nurse go from patient to patient efficiently, leaving them better off? Study what they are doing and do more of it. Keep in mind as you assess your current processes and staff that sometimes people who seem the least busy have found the most efficient way to get something done.

Teaming Up for Better Flow

After monitoring the matching and mismatching of demand and capacity and forecasting who's going to come to your ED, how many will come, and when, you may be tempted to increase the size of your staff. We've already noted that doing so will not necessarily improve flow in your ED. If you need to be convinced, consider that one study of a number of hospitals found that those with the largest staffs had the slowest throughput of patients. This result may reflect a tendency of a large staff to spend more time interacting and less time processing patients.

Certainly, a staff too small to handle the patient flow effectively will not move patients through with timely, quality care either. In our experience working with hospitals, we have found that the size of the staff is generally not the most important factor in attaining effective flow. How well the team performs is much more critical in meeting ED goals.

To improve flow, training your staff to work together well as a team is one of the best steps you can take, and it relates to many of your other efforts to smooth flow. Good teamwork can help eliminate waste. We define waste as anything that does not add value to the system. Often, waste involves duplication of effort. Is the patient getting both a triage assessment and then a nursing assessment? How many times is the patient asked to supply his or her name? Waste can also involve unnecessary delays because of department processes. Is information getting to the right staff members without wasted time? For example, an x-ray technician takes an x-ray. The patient returns to the room and waits. The doctor does not know that the x-ray has been done. That unit of time is a waste. Making simple changes to coordinate work as a team eliminates waste. One hospital laminated index cards with "x-ray back" written on them and had an x-ray technician place one on the patient's chart and then put the chart in the physician's action box, thus eliminating the wasted time. Doing so increased throughput of patients with x-rays by 15–45 minutes. You need to examine every step of every process to find and eliminate activities that do not add value.

Now let's examine some practical methods to smooth flow in your ED. As you consider the following tools, keep an underlying concept in mind: Teamwork is critical.

Tools for Smoothing Flow

One concept to keep patients flowing smoothly through your ED is parallel streams. You need to treat patients with different needs simultaneously rather than sequentially. To do so, you'll want to separate patients into different streams. You distinguish patients with different needs in several ways. The simplest involves classifying them into two groups.

The two-dimensional department

When you hear "two dimensions," what often springs to mind, especially in relation to geometry, are vertical and horizontal. These dimensions apply in the ED, as well. They're the most basic distinction between patients coming into your department. Vertical patients are just that—they walk in on their own. Horizontal patients are carried in. Generally, vertical patients are not very sick, whereas horizontal patients are really sick. There are exceptions, of course, which is why you need more than this two-dimensional way of categorizing patients. But for the most part, distinguishing vertical from horizontal patients is a useful way to start.

Vertical patients have the lowest satisfaction, which may not be too surprising. If you treat patients sequentially rather than sorting them into streams for parallel treatment, the walking wounded will often wait the longest for treatment, while more urgent cases take priority. Because they are not seriously ill, they value speed, convenience, and cost. They should get a focused evaluation and treatment and then be released. Both effective treatment of these patients and effective flow in your ED are enhanced by sorting incoming patients and routing these vertical ones through a system designed to handle them quickly and efficiently.

Horizontal patients are less concerned with convenience, speed, and cost. Their focus is strongly on one thought: "Am I going to live?" They usually will need a bed.

Vertical patients, on the other hand, generally will not need a bed. Here is where the Theory of Constraints applies: If your number of beds is likely to become a bottleneck, the more vertical patients you can keep out of beds, the better you manage that bottleneck. Most EDs send every patient to a room, where they stay until they are finished in the ED. Not only is this pattern not the best model, it is also ineffective. Unless there is a specific reason for a patient to be in a bed, then that patient should not be in one.

Flowing in four streams

There are always exceptions to the vertical–horizontal rule. As a result, we can define patient types more accurately by distinguishing the following four streams coming into the ED:

- Patients who need minor urgent care

- Trauma patients and others who need critical care

- Patients who need treatment and release

- Patients who need treatment and admission

Sorting patients in this way helps you more efficiently direct them on the path to the most effective treatment and smoothest flow (Figure 4.4). Patients in the first group have problems such as ankle sprains, foot fractures, and simple lacerations—problems that need care but are not life-threatening. These patients can be fast-tracked. Patients in the second group often have life-threatening problems. They too can be fast-tracked to a critical care unit. (Our terminology here raises a point we often make: "Fast track" is not just a noun, a place in the ED; it is also a verb, a process you follow.) Forecasting is valuable in treating this second group. If you study patterns over time, you know these patients are coming, you know when they'll arrive, and you know what their diseases are.

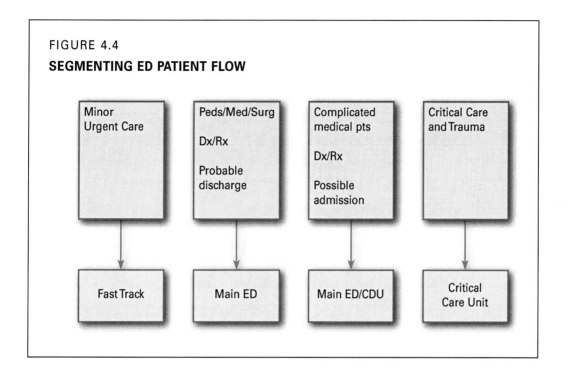

FIGURE 4.4

SEGMENTING ED PATIENT FLOW

Minor Urgent Care	Peds/Med/Surg Dx/Rx Probable discharge	Complicated medical pts Dx/Rx Possible admission	Critical Care and Trauma
Fast Track	Main ED	Main ED/CDU	Critical Care Unit

The dilemma in sorting concerns the last two groups, which constitute the middle in treatment needs between the first two. Patients in the third group need value-added services, such as lab work, x-rays, and some form of treatment. They have a 90% chance of going home after that service. Those in the fourth group need value-added services, as well, but they have a 90% chance of being admitted. The more closely you can distinguish those that fall into the 90% range in either category and route accordingly, the better flow will be in your ED.

Flowing on five levels

An even further level of sorting helps you distinguish patient types more finely. An acuity index classifies patient conditions at different levels. We can describe these in this way (and in this order, to fit our discussion):

- Level 1: Critical patients who may die unless somebody does something

- Level 5: Stable patients who may not require resources other than an encounter with a doctor or a nurse

- Level 2: High-risk patients who need multiple resources

- Level 4: Patients who need a simple x-ray, simple lab test, or simple injection

- Level 3: Patients who fall in between other levels and are tougher to treat

The majority of patients who enter your ED will fall into Level 3. As we said, they're more difficult to sort and diagnose. However, many EDs are now fast-tracking 40%–50% of Level 3 patients. The following describes how you can effectively sort these patients.

Keeping the streams flowing

As patients enter the ED, they go into triage first. The triage nurse takes their name, age, vital signs, and a cursory history and then decides where they go next. The triage nurse asks:

- Do they go in the high-acuity pathway (Levels 1 and 2)?

- Are they really sick? Do they need to go to the core area in the ED or to a bed?

- Are they Level 5 or Level 4 patients who are not too sick?

- Are they Level 3 patients who will need resources?

We can view the triage nurse as sort of the front loader for the department. The nurse can direct patients to the team triage area or have a physician see them and then send them to a fast track. Some patients can go directly to a super track or fast track for evaluation, treatment, and discharge. Other patients have lab work or an x-ray done and then go to a secondary waiting room. Still others, who are really sick, get tests done in the front of the ED but then go to the back for treatment in the core area.

Components of the ED that aid flow after triage include:

- Team triage

- Fast track

- Super track

Team triage comprises a multidisciplinary assessment and treatment team with a physician or midlevel provider, a nurse, a technician, a registrar, and a scribe (or, depending on the ED, two physicians or midlevel providers, two nurses, two scribes, and the registrar and technician). The team promptly assesses, treats, and discharges Level 3 patients. For those patients not discharged immediately, the team starts the workup and either routes those patients to a results waiting room or moves them into the fast track for further care, depending on their level of acuity. (Figure 4.5 shows a model.)

FIGURE 4.5

TEAM TRIAGE: PROMPTLY ASSESSES, TREATS, AND DISCHARGES LEVEL 3 PATIENTS

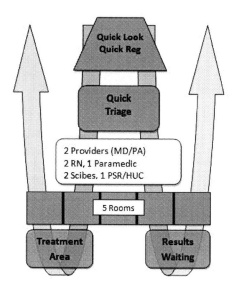

Team triage model from Mary Washington Hospital "Rated-ER" design. Courtesy of Jody Crane, MD, MBA.

The fast track's role is to segment and serve those patients who are uncomplicated or relatively easy to treat—Level 4 and 5 and some Level 3 patients. Having a fast track working at optimal speed will significantly improve your ED's performance.

The super track is a fast track located in or near triage. It typically consists of a two-bed area with a midlevel provider or a physician, a nurse, and a technician (see Figure 4.6 for an example). The super track sees Level 5 patients and some Level 4 patients whom the super-track staff can treat and discharge right away.

FIGURE 4.6

A SUPER TRACK: PROMPTLY TREAT PATIENTS WHO REQUIRE FEW RESOURCES

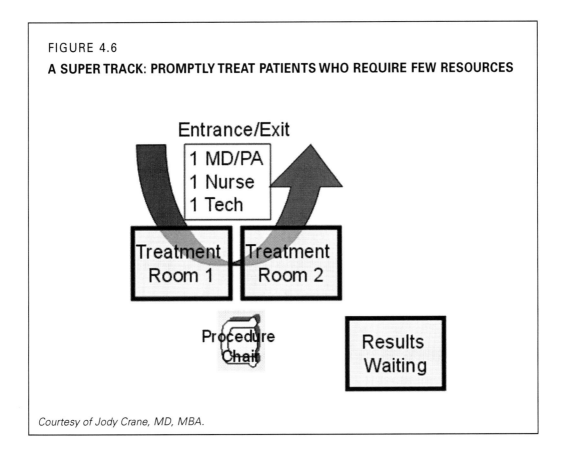

Courtesy of Jody Crane, MD, MBA.

When segmenting patient flow into streams, you design a unique way to care for each segment. Map where this design fits in your ED. Translate the concept into your setting. You need to figure out where it works in your ED, how it fits your physical layout, how it affects your culture, and whether your staff is ready for it. Don't segment your patient flow for the sake of segmenting. Narrow your streams only to the point that you can apply a different level of unique service to each.

The ED Is Not an Island

All the theories and methods we've discussed in this chapter will help speed flow, and doing so is critical to providing quality care. But we need to look beyond the ED. How we relate to other departments in the hospital affects our ability to bring significant change. Because the hospital is one system, all its departments should operate as one team, with the same goal: delivering quality care to patients. ED staff members are so accustomed to taking on problems that it does not occur to us that other departments should handle some of them. If you have a patient bound for the ICU boarding in the ED, you have an inpatient in an outpatient bed. That patient is a concern of the ICU, not the ED. Why is the ICU allowed to say no to caring for that patient? Are the hallways upstairs any worse than the hallways in the ED? (The answer is no.) Hospitals that operate as a single interrelated system have protocols for moving patients out of the ED into the hospital area where they belong, even when bed space is unavailable. They perceive this issue as a floor problem, not an ED problem.

The ED has input (patients arriving), throughput (patients being treated), and output (patients being admitted to the hospital or sent home). The most difficult part of improving flow is getting admitted patients into the hospital units where they belong. Most EDs admit around 20% of their patients. This percentage is significant, and it just happens to match part of the equation in Pareto's paradox, named after the nineteenth-century economist who formulated it:

Twenty percent of your work will cause 80% of your problems or occupy 80% of your time.

In the ED, that 20% waiting for admission often does cause 80% of the problems. Resolving the paradox requires applying queuing theory and reducing variability. It also often requires changes in the way an ED interacts with the rest of the hospital system in order to improve the flow for patients who need to be admitted.

Hospital personnel with a progressive vision will be essential in this process of change, especially a CEO who's committed to expediting ED admissions. In one hospital, a new chief nursing officer, whose guiding philosophy was that the hallways upstairs were just as good as the hallways downstairs and that more accurate care could be given on the floor where the patients belonged than in the generalized chaos of the ED, changed the way that hospital dealt with ED patients awaiting admission. Personnel who share a vision of the hospital working as a single entity are a critical component of an effective system.

Equally important is tracking data, not just in the ED but in the entire system. In one ED, we could not get telemetry patients and rule-outs admitted. We examined data from the cardiac department and discovered that half of their admissions clearly did not meet the standard measures established by the American College of

Cardiologists for admission to a cardiac-monitored unit. Because we had command of the data, we brought about a needed change in that area.

Admissions and bed controls

The largest percentage of admissions to the hospital arrive from the ED. The hospital's best interest is served by having an efficient ED, not only from a patient-care standpoint, but from a business perspective as well. Here are some actions that can help achieve that efficiency:

- Streamline the transfer system

- Streamline the hospital's admission and discharge processes

- Institute border patrol

- Coordinate bed management

Streamlining transfers

Examine the transfer process closely to see whether it contains redundancies, loops, or gaps in information flow. Someone in the ED—the charge nurse, ED case manager, or patient-flow coordinator—should be constantly on the alert for open beds in the hospital. If you do not have a person performing this function, the floor with an open bed may neglect to tell you that it is available, unnecessarily increasing the ED length of stay for the patient and slowing down throughput. Use data you have tracked to forecast how many beds you'll need each day. Try to have the bed coordinator allocate that number of beds to the ED ahead of time. Share predictions of discharges from the ED to inpatient units at the morning bed huddle.

Streamlining admission and discharge

Establishing a streamlined admissions process with a centralized bed authority has greatly improved flow in some hospitals we've worked with. Instead of making five phone calls and talking to three people, you get the patients admitted through a single, simple process. An appointment-based admission and discharge process is also effective. Most hospitals use a batch-and-queue system, which often creates backlogs and difficulties with time and staff management, thus resulting in overloads and long waits. Using appointments, staff members can plan for admissions and discharges. Using the data you have tracked, you might realize that the cardiac floor averages three admissions per day. If that unit sets up admissions for 10 a.m., 2 p.m., and 5 p.m. (for example), those admissions are built into the day, smoothing flow and reducing variation. Similarly, if you discharge patients at set times staggered throughout the day, then families know when to arrive, nurses can plan for discharges, and the process becomes more orderly.

Patrolling the border

The same person who oversees the transfer process should be aware of from where patients being cared for in the ED are entering the department. A few years ago, nurses in the outpatient transfusion center at a hospital were moving their patients to the ED when the patients were not ready to go home at the end of the nurses' workday—a time when the ED was getting really busy. A patient getting a blood transfusion at an outpatient center should not be finishing that process in the ED for the convenience of the center's employees. That patient is in a completely inappropriate setting, not only from a patient-care perspective, but also from a business perspective. This type of use of the ED should be eliminated. If someone provides transfusions for a living, that group needs to adjust hours and staffing to provide the service it is being paid for. The ED gains no revenue from these patients.

Coordinating bed management

Placing bed controls in the department helps with bed management in the hospital in general. The bed coordinator for the hospital should know the overall flow of the hospital well and should decide where patients go who are being admitted. In addition, a committee should huddle twice per day to coordinate effective patient placement. People involved in bed management should carry out triage throughout the system. For example, meet at night and examine who in the ICU can move. In the hospital as a whole, who can move? Who can be discharged? Who is in the appropriate place—or not? Coordinate with the house staff members so that you are informed when a bed is available.

Flow in the ED: A Final Look

Various methods exist to implement flow-improvement processes. The following are some of the better-known ones:

- Lean

- Rapid-cycle testing

- Six Sigma

- Total quality management

- Statistical process control

Pick one or any combination. These toolkits are immensely useful, but they are not solutions in themselves. If you can get most of your people who are actually working in the system to have some sort of rudimentary understanding of these principles, it is amazing how far you can go, because your people will create the improvements that you need.

When you start working to improve flow, set a goal for moving patients through the ED. In our studies, the best-practicing departments got their patients out in 43 minutes; the worst took 118 minutes. Your goal might be to get your patients out of the ED within, say, 60 minutes 80% of the time. Then set up a process and monitor it to make sure people are adhering to it.

As you work to improve flow, keep the following principles in mind:

- Flow is a complex, technical problem

- Flow cannot be solved by one department

- Improving flow requires high levels of cooperation and integration across multiple departments

- Smooth patient flow cannot be installed, layered on, or mandated by management

- Improving flow requires effective diagnosis of the problems and then testing of changes using multiple "plan, do, study, act" cycles

- Improving flow means changing a culture, not just a process

CASE STUDY

Physicians in triage

The situation

Two hospitals were suffering from:

- Door-to-doctor delays

- Reduced patient satisfaction, particularly in regard to timeliness and physicians being informative

- Slower-than-benchmark treat-and-release lengths of stay (LOS)

The background

ED A is a rural West Virginia hospital that treated 42,000 patients in 2007, and it admits 20% of its patient visits.

ED B is located in suburban Chicago and treated 72,000 patients in 2007. It has a distinct six-bed pediatric ED that treated 9,000 patients. It admits 30% of its nonpediatric patient visits.

Both hospitals have been ineffective at expediting care for patients with moderate to low acuity levels. Level 4 patients are those who need a simple x-ray, lab test, or injection. Level 5 patients are stable and may not require resources other than an encounter with a doctor or a nurse.

Both EDs have significant admission boarding problems as well.

CASE STUDY

Physicians in triage (cont.)

What we did

We conducted trials of eight shifts in one calendar month at each hospital. Each trial placed a physician in the triage unit to oversee, supervise, and participate in facilitating the triage process, while also treating and discharging Level 4 and 5 patients who could be segmented out of the flow before entering the rest of the ED. Five-question satisfaction surveys were verbally administered at time of discharge by the discharge nurse.

Our findings and conclusions

ED A achieved significant improvement in lower-acuity patient LOS, patient satisfaction, and reduction of door-to-doctor time.

ED B achieved improvement in lower-acuity patient LOS and door-to-doctor time. Patient satisfaction data were not consistently collected in order to yield valid findings.

Lessons

- Study patient arrival by hour of the day and day of the week if daily arrivals vary by more than 10%. Confirm that there is sufficient Level 4 and 5 patient volume to achieve three patients per hour. (In the case of ED B, the pediatric ED segmented roughly 25 Level 4 and 5 patients, thus making the pool of less-acute patients more limited.)

Physicians in triage (cont.)

- Determine on which level three patients' treatment may be started in triage and what volume it may represent.

- Consider using scribes to assist the physician in order to achieve at least three patients per hour.

	Pre		Trial	
	A	B	A	B
Total LOS (minutes)	240	260	235	240
Treat-and-release LOS (minutes)	190	195	90	105
Average number of patients treated per hour	1.7	1.5	2.8	2.0
Patient satisfaction (percentile)	30	45	95	NA

CASE STUDY

Poor performance in the fast track

The background

A central North Carolina hospital with 45,000 annual ED visits was running a 15-hour-per-day fast track staffed by midlevel providers. The average treat-and-release turn-around time of the fast track exceeded 180 minutes, and patient satisfaction scores from patients receiving services in the fast track were below the 10th percentile among Press Ganey's ED benchmark comparative group.

What we did

We engaged help from North Carolina Industrial Extension Service consultants to help with a flow-mapping consultation with ED leadership—the medical director, the nurse director, and others as needed. The goal of the process flow mapping was to identify constraints and opportunities to reduce throughput time and to engage the clinician and nursing staff so the fast track would be a center of excellence in service and performance.

At the same time, the associate medical director mentored the midlevel providers about the Press Ganey survey questions, expectations, and techniques for improving the patient interaction.

The results

The following graph displays fast-track Press Ganey score improvement. Unfortunately, the super-track plan was never fully deployed due to staffing constraints. It was clearly believed that implementation of the super-track concept could have reduced throughput time significantly, segmented Level 4 and 5 patients as well as certain patient clinical

Poor performance in the fast track (cont.)

categories of Level 3 patients, and resulted in 35% of the daily patient visits being segmented and processed through the fast/super track.

Fast track					
	May	April	March	February	January
Standard doctors	84.6	77.3	74.4	75.3	76.2
Courtesy	86.5	80.1	78.3	79.3	82.1
Time to listen	84.6	76.3	74.1	74.4	76.0
Informative retreatment	84.6	76.3	72.2	74.4	70.8
Concern for comfort	82.2	75.7	73.1	74.4	74.5

References

1. Roberts, A. Masters and Commanders: How Four Titans Won the War in the West 1941-45. New York: HarperCollins, 2009.

2. Ibid.

Ensuring Patient Satisfaction

If you're like most people, you have on occasion experienced remarkable customer service. Unfortunately, you probably remember your experiences of poor customer service much more clearly. People talk five times more frequently about poor experiences than favorable ones. But they will talk about a positive experience. Patients who encounter a problem during their ED visit that might cause them to complain later will most likely be satisfied if the problem is resolved on the spot. They'll also be surprised, which is why 95% of them will tell others about that positive experience. The difference between those patients—or customers—who are satisfied with their care in your ED and those who are not is a critical indicator of how effectively your department carries out its mission. Consider the following customer service experience.

My two-year-old digital camera stopped working properly. I assumed that repairing the camera would cost more than buying a new one. I also doubted I would find anyone who could repair it in the first place. Nonetheless, I decided to visit the camera company's website. I learned there that the company fully supports all of its cameras. I was directed to call the company's service center. A live person answered my call on the second ring and asked my name, telephone number, and the model of my camera and then transferred me directly to a service technician. The technician confirmed the information I had provided to the first caller— without requiring me to repeat it—and got my e-mail address in order to send me mailing instructions and a printable return address label. The technician then described three things:

- What the service process entails

- The normal time servicing takes

- Potential outcomes of servicing

That same day, the technician's e-mail arrived, along with the mailing instructions, the return label, and an invoice for the service fee. The e-mail also repeated the points the technician had made during the call.

I returned the camera along with a $15 check for the fee. Five days before the projected return date, I got my repaired camera, along with a 30-day warranty. Soon after it arrived, the technician called to make sure the camera worked and asked if I had any questions or concerns. I was impressed by the whole experience.

The following is what made this experience so outstanding:

- **Courtesy:** I was treated professionally, courteously, efficiently, and expeditiously. The company's representatives valued my time; the technician not only achieved but bettered the time commitment made.

- **Listening:** Both the operator and the service technician listened to me carefully to determine what was wrong and what steps they should follow.

- **Informing:** Both the operator and technician gave understandable expectations of servicing. The technician explained the servicing process verbally and summarized it in the e-mail. I was kept informed and knew what to expect.

- **Concern:** The camera worked after the servicing, and an added benefit, of which I wasn't aware, was that the repairs were warranted. The same technician who took my original inquiry followed up with me to close the customer interaction loop.

Now ask yourself how well your staff does this with each patient in your ED. They are, after all, your customers. Doing everything you can to ensure that they are happy with the service you are providing is critical to implementing the improvement project for your ED. When your patients are not happy, your hospital will suffer. The following describes how we can measure it.

The Cost of Dissatisfied Patients

No one likes to hear complaints about the service they provide. But as much as you don't like to hear complaints, you should remember that the vast majority of dissatisfied customers never complain. A complaint reveals only the tip of the iceberg. Each patient who is unhappy with the service in your ED and complains represents six other patients who were equally disappointed. Even though they may not complain to you, you can bet they will complain to other people; typically, they relate the experience to eight to 10 other people. Now you have roughly 63 people who have heard about the negative encounter. As a result, about one in four will decide not to come to your ED if they need treatment. At an average revenue of $500 per visit and an average of five lifetime visits per patient, the total revenue lost from these 16 patients is $40,000. And that's just for one complaint.

But you're not done losing money yet. When a patient complains, you have to handle that complaint, which entails costs. The average ED complaint requires $375 in costs to the department. For a department with an average number of complaints—around 52 per year—the cost of dealing with these complaints amounts to $19,500 annually.

If you want to keep treating patients, you need to figure out ways to keep them happy.

History of healthcare service

When prospective healthcare administrators trained 25 years ago, they learned five primary characteristics to consider when evaluating healthcare service:

1. Access to care

2. Continuity of care

3. Comprehensiveness of care

4. Quality of care

5. Cost effectiveness of care

What's not in that list? Customer service. At that time, the term *customer* was never even uttered, because healthcare professionals believed it would denigrate the patient relationship. Patient satisfaction, if considered at all, was subsumed under quality of care. Times have changed.

If you analyze that list in the context of the ED, customer satisfaction rises even higher on it now than it has risen in many other areas. The obvious component in access to care—being able to reach a facility that provides emergency care—is available for most people. Another part of access, and a characteristic that was considered 25 years ago, is choice—the ability to choose between different facilities. How many individuals wake up in the morning and set this goal: My day will be fulfilled if I achieve a visit to the ED? People usually end up in the ED because of circumstances beyond their control. Access to care, in the sense of choice, is in effect moot in regard to emergency care. Continuity of care, while obviously very important, is usually more of a factor beyond the ED when patients transfer. Comprehensiveness of care involves coordination of healthcare professional team members' efforts within the department. It's a critical factor. However, coordination goes on mostly behind the scenes. And to the extent that patients notice, it is closely related to their perception of customer service—positive or negative.

Clearly, quality is essential, and it is tied closely with patients' perception of customer service. Cost effectiveness is often masked from patients during their visits, largely because of statutes requiring that a medical evaluation be provided to any patient presenting in an ED and because relatively few hospitals actively pursue collection of copays or deductibles during the visit.

In the past quarter-century, more emphasis has been placed on healthcare professionals being attuned to and proactively seeking to improve the patient's satisfaction when providing healthcare. Increasingly, this emphasis has been driven by economic reasons, by regulatory agencies imposing minimally accepted standards of service, and by consumers themselves who demand better service and who have more information about healthcare conditions immediately accessible, especially from the Internet, than in years past. As a result, hospital trustees often incorporate patient-satisfaction goals in healthcare executives' bonus criteria. Healthcare administrators must focus on customer satisfaction to remain competitive. And the ED as the front door of the hospital is a visible arena, where customer satisfaction or dissatisfaction significantly affects community perception about the quality of the hospital as a whole.

Competition and consumer demand are among the primary differences in how we evaluated healthcare services 25 years ago and how we do so today. (See Figure 5.1 for these differences.)

FIGURE 5.1

CHANGES IN EVALUATING PROVISION OF HEALTHCARE SINCE 1985

25 Years Ago	Now
Medical staff (private attending physicians) generates ≥ 75% of hospital admissions	Emergency departments often generate ≥ 75% of hospital inpatient admissions (private attending physicians opt to have hospitalists provide inpatient care)
Very little competition	Tremendous competition (both from other providers and ever increasingly from financial pressures to remain viable)
Managed care payers or payer contracts do not define care standards	Payer agreements define specific care standards and impose penalties for not meeting care standards (customer satisfaction components included)
Physician identified as the primary customer	Physician shares the identity of primary customer with patient and payer

Improving Patient Satisfaction

The following are four steps to raise the satisfaction of your customers:

- Reduce wait times

- Make structural changes

- Manage perceptions and expectations

- Analyze patient-satisfaction surveys and complaints

We often equate customer service to just being nice rather than making a deep exploration into what the customer values in the ED entail. For example, structural change refers to improving the cleanliness and the appearance of the waiting room, ensuring privacy in the registration area, making blankets and pillows available, and providing comfortable chairs. You need to really analyze surveys and complaints to identify factors that lead to patient satisfaction or the lack thereof. Most departments simply respond to particular survey points rather than embed customer satisfaction as an integral part of their ED processes.

Ask the patients—and tell the doctors

EDs are different than, say, a restaurant because they are held accountable for excellent patient satisfaction by customers who don't want to be there. Most hospitals survey their patients to gauge the extent to which desired attributes of patient satisfaction were present, as well as patients' overall perception of their experience. What do these surveys ask patients, and does your staff know what patients are grading them on? Is your staff aware of the survey results? We have

  The Hospital Executive's Guide to Emergency Department Management

consulted with hospitals throughout the United States, and we are continually surprised at how few physicians and nurses have seen an actual copy of the patient-satisfaction survey upon which their performance is judged. The survey should be an open-book test, and all professionals involved in providing care in the ED should know what questions the patient will be asked. Besides providing your team a copy of the survey, you should also hold discussion and coaching sessions and coordinate these activities so the team can focus its efforts on those characteristics that will improve a patient's experience. Remember our example of camera repair and how communication, including expectations, and minimal handoffs were well coordinated.

Patient-satisfaction surveys tend to boil down to questions covering the following four main topics:

- Courtesy

- How much time the staff took to listen to the patient

- How well informed the patient was about the treatment

- The doctor's concern about the patient's comfort

Do these have a familiar ring? EDs may have an unusual context for expectations of customer service, but they are essentially the same as our reflections on why the camera repair experience was positive. Keep that example in mind as we look at these four themes in emergency care. (We'll use doctors in our discussion, but it applies to nurses and other staff members on the healthcare team as well).

Courtesy of the staff

Courtesy is a fundamental component of effective human communication. Verbal aspects of interaction between healthcare providers and patients demonstrate the truth of this assertion. However, nonverbal behavior is also significant. If the patient observes the physician looking at the clock or a wristwatch, the patient forms an impression of his or her relative importance to the physician, and it probably won't result in the patient rating the doctor's courtesy highly. Administrators should help doctors see how they're perceived by sharing comments from patients on surveys that offer insight on the interactions. The more closely the comments can be tied to real interactions with actual patients, allowing doctors to re-create the interaction, the more beneficial this sharing will be.

Taking time to listen

The patient's perception of this characteristic depends not only on the actual time spent in the interaction but in the quality of the communication. Once again, nonverbal behavior plays a crucial role in forming the patient's perception about how much time the doctor took to listen. If the doctor sits down when speaking with the patient, then the perception is usually that the doctor has taken more time even if the actual duration isn't any different than if the doctor had remained standing. How involved the patient is allowed to be in the conversation is another important factor in the patient's perception of how well the doctor listened. Remember that perception forms not just from the actual duration of time spent, but also from the content of the communication.

Informing the patient

How well informed the patient feels depends not only on what information the doctor provides, but also in how the doctor provides it. Did the physician include expectations of how the treatment will proceed and what it will accomplish? How other members of the healthcare team reinforce this information also helps determine the patient's perception. Informing the patient is a challenge to many healthcare professionals, because of the barriers erected by the use of medical terminology—acronyms, abbreviations, and "medicalese" in general. Hospitals, in this regard, are often not user-friendly to the public.

Concern for comfort

People don't go to the ED unless they have to, and pain is usually the reason patients are there. A key part of the patient's perception about the quality of treatment is how well the doctor or nurse understands his or her level of pain and how adequately the team member responds to ameliorate it. Patients need to feel heard, need to understand the process for assessing their condition, and need to understand what latitude the doctor has to reduce their pain.

Techniques to Satisfy Your Patients

We recommend a couple approaches to address patients' overall satisfaction with their experience in your ED, and thus their likelihood of recommending your ED to others. One is the set of techniques incorporated in our Survival Skills© training course to recruit for customer service skills, teach actions that lead to excellent customer service, track patient-satisfaction scores, tailor coaching to specific results for specific individuals, and analyze team behaviors. Another approach is the use of scripts. These contain specific wording intended to address the patients' concerns we've been discussing. Often, more-experienced doctors, nurses, and other team members can provide the content to less-experienced professionals. Contributing to an overall impression of care are the following behaviors:

- Complete explanations

- Promptness

- Friendliness and caring

- Putting patients at ease

- Providing updates and feedback

The patient's experience begins when that person arrives at the ED, and the factors involved in creating satisfaction start at that moment: the wait time before the patient's arrival is noticed, helpfulness of the first person encountered, and comfort of the waiting area, followed by the wait time to reach the treatment area and then the wait time to see the doctor. Actions you can take that lead to a satisfying encounter during these initials stages are to keep the reception and waiting areas clean; provide frequent updates; set expectations for the patient early; offer diversions in the waiting room for all age groups, including a play area for young children, health-network television, and educational materials; post or otherwise communicate waiting times; establish a separate entrance and waiting area for fast-track patients; provide coffee for families of patients who face long stays in the ED; and have patient associates who communicate with waiting family members and a customer service representative who makes rounds in the waiting room.

You should drill into your staff's consciousness this goal: Door-to-doctor time should be 25 minutes 60% of the time.

Another aspect of the initial stages that impacts the patient's sense of satisfaction is taking personal insurance information down. It is important to treat patients with courtesy and provide them privacy during the collection of this information. The ease of giving this information is also important.

After that introductory phase, initial contact between team members and the patient forms the all-important first impression of the treatment process. Your doctors, nurses, and other professionals should practice the following behaviors that reinforce the positive tone you should already have established in the first phase, such as:

- Knock before entering

- Recognize the patient's concern about time

- Thank the patient for waiting

- Introduce yourself to everyone in the room

- Acknowledge the patient's concerns

- Demonstrate caring and respect for privacy

- Explain transitions

The closing phase of the patient's encounter is just as important as the initial greeting. Make sure the discharge process is simple and understandable. Coach staff members to use scripts to clarify expectations of service in this process and resolve problems.

Getting to know the staff

You shouldn't underestimate the importance of setting the right tone from the beginning. But the central phase that establishes the conditions for satisfying patients is the behavior of your healthcare professionals in treating them. For physicians, the key aspects are the doctor's courtesy, whether the doctor took time to listen and informed the patient what to expect with treatment, and the doctor's concern for the patient's comfort. Coach your doctors to keep the patients informed, introduce themselves properly, sit with the patients whenever possible, conduct an exit visit whenever possible, use scripts, and attend to the patient's pain and general comfort.

For nurses, the expectations are similar and include their courtesy to patients and their families and friends, whether they took time to listen and inform patients and their families and friends, their attention to patients' needs, their concern for privacy, and whether they let family and friends stay with patients. Train and mentor your nurses in how to use scripts, be aware of comfort and caring concerns, frequently contact patients and families and explain treatment and transitions, check in every hour to see whether they need blankets and pillows, and make contact every 15–30 minutes.

In regard to your technicians as well as nurses, significant factors are the courtesy of the person who draws blood and concern over the patient's comfort during this procedure, wait time for radiology tests, courtesy of the radiology staff, and concern for comfort during those tests.

Doctors, nurses, and administrators should also be visible to patients. You can do this by conducting regularly scheduled rounds to observe and reinforce behavior.

Helping to resolve problems as they're occurring is also important for management. Staff members should be trained to resolve problems while they're occurring by rehearsing potential situations. Providing buttons to staff members that read "Ask me" or "May I help you?" and business cards are simple tools that help reinforce your staff members' efforts to satisfy their patients. Administrators should ensure that there is follow-up contact by phone for every patient who leaves the ED against medical advice or leaves without being seen and for every pediatric patient within 24 hours.

Senior leaders should also track patient-satisfaction scores, compliments, and complaints by provider. Celebrate accomplishments in customer service. Train staff members in survival skills and reinforce them. Selectively use secret shoppers to test the quality of customer service in your ED. Conduct patient focus groups.

Management should be sensitive to the satisfaction not just of patients but of another group as well: attending staff members—both internal and external. Hold regular meetings—one to five per month—and encourage committee participation, including that of the executive committee. You should also conduct satisfaction surveys of attending staff members.

Overall issues of quality

Consider specific methods to enhance customer satisfaction during various phases of treatment, but make sure that you reinforce key behaviors that staff members should always practice with patients regardless of the patients' stage of treatment and passage through the ED. These include providing complete explanations; being prompt, friendly, and caring; putting patients at ease; and providing updates and feedback.

Remember that patients always want to be informed about delays throughout their entire ED encounter. They want to feel like the staff members care about them as people, and they want to have their pain controlled. They want to receive information about home care that they understand, and they want to feel safe in the hospital.

PATIENT WAITING

One experience we all share much too often in modern life is waiting in line. The psychology of waiting concerns how we perceive different aspects of that experience. From studies delving into the psychology of waiting, organizations have developed methods to manage waits and to exploit the findings about our perceptions of waiting. Businesses, in particular, have made good use of those methods. When you are unable to avoid a queue, understanding the principles derived from the studies and applying the resulting methods help enhance patients' perceptions of flow and thus increase patient satisfaction. In a sense, you're inducing artificial flow—but doing so is okay in this context. There is a lot of material available on the psychology of waiting (see *Leadership for Smooth Patient Flow* and *Hardwiring Flow: Systems and Processes for Seamless Patient Care*).[1, 2] The following are some of the principles first identified by David Maister in 1984.[3]

Time with nothing to do seems longer

When you're behind two grocery carts loaded with items at the checkout counter, time seems to drag forever. You have nothing to do other than stare at the candy or tabloids. If, on the other hand, you've ever been in line at the Star Tours ride at Disney World, you probably recall winding your way through a building with androids in various states of repair, exotic machines, and realistic props, creating the impression that you're inside an enormous hangar in the *Star Wars* galaxy and leaving you so absorbed that you may actually regret moving too fast past some props. You may actually wait 15 minutes in the grocery line and 30 minutes in the Disney queue, but the former seems twice as long as the latter. To take a simpler example, restaurants often provide waiting customers with menus to look over before their table is ready or direct them to the bar, where there is usually a television with sporting events on. We tend to perceive waiting when we have nothing to occupy the time as dragging on longer than when we can concentrate on something interesting.

PATIENT WAITING (CONT.)

We can put the same principle to work in EDs. Providing magazines to read and a television to watch gives patients something to do while they wait. Filling out necessary forms as part of registration does too. The more patients perceive that they have something interesting to do to pass the time while they're waiting, the more satisfied they'll be. Allowing them to have family members or friends wait with them helps them pass the time more pleasantly.

A similar perception makes us think that if we get started in an activity quickly, the entire activity goes more quickly than when we have to wait longer to begin, even if the overall time spent in the activity is similar. We can take advantage of this perception in the ED by using tools that improve flow anyway, such as triage, team triage, and sending patients directly to a room. You keep patient satisfaction high while you smooth flow. Moving patients sequentially also gives them a sense that they are in process, so if patients go from triage to registration to a room, the time seems to pass more quickly than if they're just waiting in the entrance area to be seen by anyone.

Uncertainty makes waiting seem longer

If your flight has been delayed and you start to worry about making a connection, you can get pretty anxious. Having to wait increases that anxiety. Uncertainty about how long you're going to have to wait makes time seem to drag as well. And unexplained delays also create the perception of time dragging. If a representative of the airline tells you what caused the delay of your flight and when you're likely to be able to leave, your anxiety level goes down. Patients encountering delays often get anxious too, and the principle for responding to that anxiety is the same: Let your patients know why delays have occurred. Regular contact with waiting patients eases their anxiety and makes the time seem to pass more quickly. Letting your patients know when they're likely to be treated and what the process will consist of provides more

PATIENT WAITING (CONT.)

certainty, which in turn helps patients' perception of time passing. If a major trauma case is occupying multiple resources, explaining why patients are waiting longer helps manage perception. Most people are likely to understand when you explain delays to them in this kind of situation.

Fairness and value

If someone cuts in the grocery line in front of you, that action triggers your sense of injustice. And when you feel your wait is unfair, it seems longer. Be aware of this perception in designing your processes and the layout of your ED. The farther apart you can keep different groups of people likely to proceed at different speeds through the department, the better you'll be able to maintain patient satisfaction. If someone waiting sees someone else who entered the ED later headed to the fast track, that person is likely to have a perception of inequitable treatment. Communication is important here, too; the more you communicate with waiting patients, explaining why someone else went ahead, the better you can manage these perceptions.

Other perceptions arise from a sense of value. If you get on the waiting list for dinner at an exclusive restaurant known for its great cuisine, waiting an hour for a table may seem a small inconvenience and well worth enduring. Waiting an hour at your ordinary neighborhood burger joint, on the other hand, is likely time you're not willing to spend. The healthcare system is no different from restaurants in this regard. If your ED has a reputation as the best in the area, with excellent care and customer service, patients will very likely submit to waiting longer without complaint. People are willing to wait longer if they perceive quality to be high. You want to enhance flow, of course, so waiting is minimized, but achieving excellence in many aspects reinforces the quality and effectiveness of all aspects of your operation.

PATIENT WAITING (CONT.)

Keeping company

If you've ever waited by yourself for an appointment, say for a job interview, you know that time spent waiting can really seem to drag. If you're waiting in a public area and end up talking with the people around you, the time seems to pass more quickly. In the ED, you can manage this perception by making sure patients can wait with family members or friends. Regular contact helps mitigate the perception of time dragging as well. If you are communicating regularly with patients who are waiting, those waiting by themselves will feel less isolated. If you can figure out how to make the general atmosphere in the waiting areas of your ED enhance communication between strangers, you'll help reduce the sense of waiting alone and thus help make the passage of time seem shorter.

References

1. Jensen, K., Mayer, T., Welch, S., Haraden, C. Leadership for Smooth Patient Flow., Chicago: Health Administration Press, 2007.

2. Mayer, T., Jensen, K. Hardwiring Flow: Systems and Processes for Seamless Patient Care. Gulf Breeze, FL: Fire Starter Publishing, 2009.

3. Maister, D. The Psychology of Waiting Lines. Harvard Business Online, April 1984.

It Takes a Team

The emergency physician is the most visible member of the staff to patients. The physicians also lead the efforts of all the staff members involved in treating your patients. The physicians may set the tone and can make a huge impact in assisting the rest of the staff, but they can't do it all themselves. Remember that the group treating your patients is a team, and achieving high levels of patient satisfaction requires that your staff functions effectively as a team. The behavior of the physician influences how well your team will work. The doctor has the opportunity to lead a winning team through winning behavior. But the doctor can also set a sour tone for the rest of the team that becomes hard to overcome. If the doctor is not effectively setting the right tone, the rest of the team will have great difficulty overcoming that poor attitude. On the other hand, if the entire team works in a well-coordinated fashion in which roles and responsibilities are well defined and the team has a shared commitment to helping each patient efficiently, effectively, and in a caring, courteous fashion, patients get better treatment and the people caring for the patients receive additional rewards for a job well done.

EDs face additional challenges beyond having customers who don't want to be there. Today, many hospitals routinely contract with management and staffing companies to provide emergency professional services. So not only are EDs challenged by having customers who don't want to be there, but the medical staff doesn't own the service. That is why involving the emergency physician group in patient-satisfaction efforts is vital. It helps ensure smooth collaboration between the physician group and the nurses. To achieve that smooth collaboration requires you and your team members to recognize the symbiotic nature of the relationship between physicians and nurses in the ED.

It also requires everyone—leadership, physicians, and staff members—to remember that your patient is a customer and you are providing that customer with a service. If your customers are not satisfied, they'll go elsewhere. But if your customers are satisfied, then your team will be too.

CASE
STUDY
A patient-satisfaction action plan

The background

Patient-satisfaction results in a central North Carolina hospital with 45,000 annual visits in the ED were consistently below the 30th percentile of Press Ganey's ED benchmark comparative group. A new administration in the hospital directed the emergency services contract group to focus additional effort on improving patient-satisfaction scores. It is important to note that scores in the fast track, which historically are higher than the main room, were significantly lower and, in fact, in single digits.

What we did

The ED leadership, which included the medical director, associate medical director, and nursing director, embarked on a 90-day initiative to achieve at least the 50th percentile rank among the Press Ganey greater-than-40,000-annual-visits ED benchmark comparative group. The initiatives included:

- Providing ED staff members with the A Team toolkit material/behaviors for review, study, and adoption

- Presenting BestPractices' Survivor Skills to hospital medical staff members

- Making Survival Skills PowerPoint® presentations and white papers available for all nursing and support staff members

- Distributing Press Ganey surveys, survey results, and scripts to all ED staff members within services to review concepts, pertinent points, and how to put them into action

CASE STUDY

A patient-satisfaction action plan (cont.)

- Conducting webinars with the entire staff to review patient-satisfaction turn-around examples

- Hiring a greeter for the ED waiting room to welcome patients' family members, ensure that their primary needs are met, update them regarding wait times, and distribute pamphlets outlining the ED process and expectations

- Implementing a patient-callback system that focuses on fast-track patients and identifying opportunities to improve fast-track turnaround

The results

The graph on the next page demonstrates improvement in both the main room and the fast-track area (see Figure 5.2). Additionally, the midlevel providers who staff the fast track were included in a bonus incentive that was shared when the overall fast-track scores exceeded the 75th percentile (see Figure 5.3).

CASE STUDY

A patient-satisfaction action plan (cont.)

FIGURE 5.2

PATIENT SATISFACTION SCORES

Emergency Department

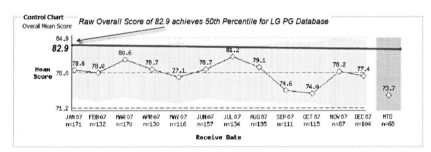

Emergency Department—Fast Track

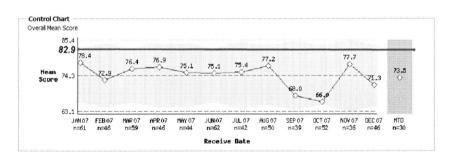

A patient-satisfaction action plan (cont.)

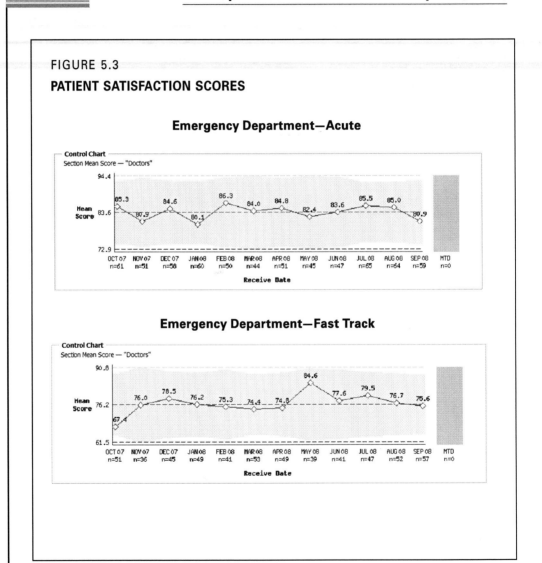

FIGURE 5.3
PATIENT SATISFACTION SCORES

Emergency Department—Acute

Emergency Department—Fast Track

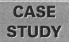

Patient-satisfaction improvement

The situation

Historically, a rural ED in central Pennsylvania with more than 50,000 annual visits performed well to very well on a locally developed patient-satisfaction survey tool. Once every two years, the organization contracted with Press Ganey to survey patients to validate the local survey results. The Press Ganey results for three quarters in 2008 and 2009 demonstrated poor to very poor performance related to ED patient satisfaction. The ED leadership team (clinicians and nursing staff members) were enlisted to improve scores.

The background

The nursing and doctor components of the scores were under the 20th percentile for the large Press Ganey database (see Figure 5.4 for baseline data).

FIGURE 5.4

PATIENT SATISFACTION SURVEY RESULTS (PRESS GANEY)

July 2008 through March 2009			
	July–September 2008	October–December 2008	January–March 2009
Likelihood to recommend (mean)	74.2	78.8	80
Standard overall (mean)	80.7	83.4	83.1
Doctor overall (mean)	81.1	85.4	85.5
Nursing overall (mean)	84.9	86.9	85.8

Patient-satisfaction improvement (cont.)

What we did:

The ED embarked on a departmentwide effort to promote awareness, solicit participation, and promote improvement. The clinician staff, through the ambulatory department committee meetings, established a seven-point plan:

1. The clinician staff was educated:

   - An introductory letter was sent to providers outlining full commitment from the top down.

   - A department meeting presentation was given by the medical director and chief medical officer.

   - Press Ganey results and survey questions were distributed to all clinicians, along with Press Ganey scripts for each primary area. The BestPractices A Team toolkit was reviewed with all clinicians.

   - A webinar to discuss the A Team toolkit and a case example was scheduled.

2. Individual discussions were conducted between each ED clinician and medical director.

3. A system for handing out business cards at each visit by the clinician was agreed upon.

4. A callback system was implemented.

5. A BestPractices Survival Skills presentation was scheduled for the entire organization.

CASE STUDY

Patient-satisfaction improvement (cont.)

6. Nurses began assessing service at discharge.

7. A plan to validate clinician-specific Press Ganey results was implemented.

FIGURE 5.5

PATIENT SATISFACTION RESULTS

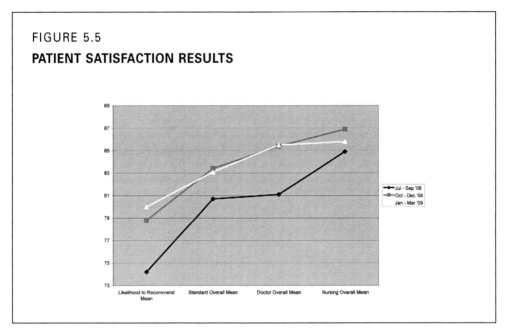

The results

The graphs in Figure 5.5 depict steady and strong improvement, particularly in the nursing score, doctor score, and willingness to recommend service at the ED. This project was implemented in a nine-month time frame, and positive results began after the first quarter.

6

Implementing the Plan

You need to design how you want your ED to be and then develop a plan to make it that way. The steps described in this chapter are essential. You're not going to get where you want to go without a road map and signposts. But directions are not enough. To complete your journey, you have to drive to the destination. And the execution phase is where many projects fail.

> *"The best way to predict the future is to create it."*
>
> —Peter Drucker

Where They Go Wrong

First let's look at why so many projects do not succeed. David J. Shulkin, MD, notes 10 common reasons many efforts to improve quality in healthcare systems fail:[1]

1. Holding too many meetings

2. Placing too much emphasis on understanding processes

3. Paying insufficient attention to incentive

4. Hiring the wrong people

5. Gathering too much data

6. Failing to learn from others

7. Lacking accountability or decision-making authority

8. Creating timelines that are too long

9. Trying to do too much

10. Not knowing when to stop

Three factors govern improvement projects: will, ideas, and execution. Too often, people undertake projects with initial enthusiasm, setting out a plan and trying to achieve it, but then fail to take steps to ensure that the project proceeds smoothly. Executing it requires continuous, careful, deliberate efforts to monitor implementation and control its direction (Figure 6.1 provides a checklist for managing projects). Failing to focus on this stage is a critical error that is all too common. However, there are ways you can avoid this failure.

Project Management 101

Not only do you need different types of leaders, but you also need a couple of teams. If this variety seems to make our efforts too diffuse, rest assured that implementing an improvement project requires different, specific types of coordination if you are going to reach your goal. You need leaders with perspectives both inside and outside your improvement team. Some of the leaders may share attributes and some roles may overlap, but the various functions we highlight all need to be in place.

FIGURE 6.1

A CHECKLIST FOR MANAGING PROJECTS

Did you	Yes	No
Designate a project manager who has sufficient time?		
Assemble a core team and a project team?		
Ensure that the planned changes and goals for your project are aligned?		
Establish a formal process for reviewing progress and planning further steps?		
Discuss these points with the sponsor?		

Designate an overall project manager and a daily leader

Your project requires a manager who can devote time to it. Taking on new projects is not unusual in healthcare, and usually we work them into our existing schedule without clearing any time. However, consider that nearly two-thirds of ED directors and administrators think total quality management (TQM) programs have been ineffective, and the most common reason cited is lack of allotted time for TQM teams. Other reasons they are ineffective include lack of administrative support, training, and employee support. An improvement project of this sort is important and complex, and it carries a great potential payoff. To ensure that it succeeds, you need a leader who can allocate time specifically for managing the project. Depending on the scope of the project, this can or often should involve anywhere from 20%–25% (perhaps even more) of that leader's work time for the duration of the project.

You also should have someone down on the shop floor, so to speak, who can monitor your project to make sure changes are being implemented. This is your day-to-day leader. This leader should understand the system in detail and should have a good grasp of the impact of various changes. The day-to-day leader should also work effectively with the physicians and nurses on the improvement team and coordinate communication between the team and leadership of the system. This leader should be allowed to dedicate a minimum of 20% of work time to the project.

Sponsors and system leaders in implementation

Your sponsor is your outside leader—someone who is not a member of the team. However, the sponsor is responsible for the team's success and is accountable to the organization for the team's performance. The sponsor's role in helping the team secure resources includes:

- Ensuring that the team has sufficient time allocated for its tasks

- Ensuring that tools needed to help team members improve as the project proceeds are available to them

- Conducting monthly review meetings with the team and receiving progress reports on tests executed and data collected

If the sponsor does not come from the system's senior leadership, that person needs to be directly connected with that leadership and must have sufficient authority to obtain resources and remove barriers. Heather Kaplan, MD, of Cincinnati Children's Hospital has described details of the sponsor's role, including:[2]

- Persuading clinicians of the benefits of the project and its importance, and motivating them

- Providing a strong sense of support so the improvement team feels confident of its ability to bring change

- Ensuring that a capable leader heads the team and making sure that person has adequate time to commit

- Promoting team cohesiveness

- Ensuring that senior clinical and managerial leaders agree with the project and are involved in implementation

- Finding a strong physician advocate

- Making sure meetings run efficiently

Even though the sponsor is not on the team, he or she should attend meetings and help the team leader run the meetings effectively.

A system leader should be on the core team. This person should be a senior member of the organization who guides the project team in its overall efforts and has real authority within the system to help the team achieve its aims. (Figure 6.2 sums up some of the responsibilities these different leaders need to embrace.) Senior leadership in the organization, through the sponsor and system leader, play three important roles in your project:

- Sponsoring the team

- Creating the vision of the new system

- Fostering the necessary cooperation to achieve the organizational goals

FIGURE 6.2

A CHECKLIST FOR MANAGING PEOPLE IN A CHANGE PROCESS

Did you	Yes	No
Develop and convey a compelling message to each group in the ED of why this work is important?		
Share the project's goals and plans outside as well as inside the ED and ask for input?		
Invite people to take part in tests (i.e., find early adopters)?		
Establish a formal process for keeping everyone aware of learning and progress?		

Reaching the Goal

The core team

Your core team will have three to eight people. A local advocate should lead this core team and should be empowered to succeed. Make sure this leader has a clear understanding of the organizational goals, the project objectives, all available data, relevant tools, and the A Team on the floor. The leader should also have clearly outlined accountability, with consequences—positive and negative—and should receive continual coaching and feedback. Having a local advocate who is highly motivated to lead this core team is essential. The administrative or corporate office cannot simply impose a solution to implementation.

Members of your core team should include the system leader, project manager, and day-to-day leader. In our experience, the roles of the project manager and the day-to-day leader are often combined. This can be effective if this person has great organizational and project management skills and can focus on the day-to-day work, while keeping his or her eye on the project timelines, progress, and resource needs. We have seen these two roles combined to limit resources allocated to the project at hand and in many of these instances the project suffers. Make sure technical expertise is also represented. A technical expert knows the subject intimately and understands the processes of care. You may need to bring in an expert on performance improvement methods who can help the team determine what to measure; help design simple, effective measurement tools; and offer advice on collecting, interpreting, and displaying data. Other examples of members of the core team are department directors of the ED, nursing clinical leaders on all shifts, nurses and physicians, and directors from ancillary services, such as radiology.

You should have at least one physician and one nurse on the team. They should have good working relationships with colleagues and the day-to-day leader. They should also have a real interest in improving the system. When you form the core team, look for physicians and nurses whom others go to for advice and who are not afraid to implement change. The core team should focus on keeping the improvement project on track, coordinate implementation, and remove obstacles to success.

ESSENTIAL CHARACTERISTICS OF THE CORE TEAM

- Working knowledge of the operations to be improved

- The ability to function as a team at an accelerated pace

- Having staff time allocated by senior leadership for the project

- Being motivated and excited about change and creating a new design

- The ability to make the team's work visible to departments involved in change through sharing results, asking for input, and involving them in tests

The project team

The project improvement team involves all the key stakeholders in the process. Even though it has more members than the core team, it should not be so large that it gets in the way of effectively implementing change. The system leader guides the overall project team. This leader also ensures clear communication with the organization's senior leadership and leadership's involvement in the progress of the work. The day-to-day leader and the project manager are also on the larger team. Other members include physicians and nurses; representatives from ancillary services, such as radiology; and representatives from support services. All should have an interest in implementing change, a willingness to be coached, and the ability to perform as part of a team.

Don't overlook one other kind of potential member of the project team: your patients. They offer a different kind of technical expertise—they have experience with the system and they know intimately the needs and wishes of patients.

When you start your project, hold a kickoff meeting with the improvement team to give an overview of the improvement project. The sponsor should lead off with remarks on why the project and the team are important and how the project connects to the organization's overall goals and strategy. The sponsor should share any available data that illustrate the organization's current performance and the gap between its current performance and the goals you want your ED to achieve. The system leader or project leader should then introduce each member and describe why that person is on the team, outline his or her roles and responsibilities, present the schedule of meetings, and indicate key milestones in the project. Team members should each describe their aspirations and concerns (record both on a flip chart) and should share any stories, data, and observations on patient experiences that are relevant. The sponsor and the project leader should then sum up and close the meeting.

Methods and Pacing

Get it in writing

As you begin the project, you should set out your plan in writing. Doing so gives you a tool that will help remind you what the steps are and enable you to gauge concretely whether you're achieving them. Everyone needs to know up front what you are going to do, who is going to do it, and by when you're going to do it. The project document will help keep you on track and help ensure that everybody is on the same page from the beginning so there is a common and shared model or plan for the project scope, goals, and objectives.

Create a feedback loop

Your written plan tells you what, where, and why. A timeline adds when and by whom. A feedback loop looks at whether it happened, and if not, why? It is not about assigning blame—understanding this point is critical to maintaining morale on your team. The loop keeps the team focused on the goals. If you haven't accomplished what you intended by your target date, assess why and act to correct any problems or overcome barriers so that you can accomplish your task. When you do achieve the steps you'd planned, let everyone know about the progress and share the credit. Give team members plenty of credit when things go right. Harry Truman once observed that you can get a lot done if you don't care who gets the credit. Spread it around.

Set the tempo

As you embark on your journey of improvement, break your timeline into segments. Think in terms of 30-, 60-, and 90-day projects. Some people set out on projects of this sort with a one- or two-year timeline in mind. However, most individuals—and most teams—work better with shorter intervals for projects. Break those segments down into even smaller intervals. Have weekly timelines for each segment's steps. Accordingly, break your project into smaller subprojects in a planned sequence and with set timelines. Going about your improvement project in this way allows you to succeed 30 days at a time. This approach is a much healthier and more successful way to get the work done than to set out on one long-term plan and schedule.

Put it to the test

Flowing out of this pacing is rapid-cycle testing.[3] This testing uses a sequence called PDSA, or "plan, do, study, act." In rapid-cycle testing, you determine one objective you will test in a short-term trial. You should be able to specify what idea you're testing, why you're testing this potential change, and what your objective is (see Figure 6.3). Your planning phase involves determining the following four things:

- What needs to be done for this cycle?

- Who is responsible?

- By when is it to be done?

- Where is it to be done?

After planning comes the doing. Carry out your plan and document problems and unexpected observations. Studying means summarizing what you learned from the test. Acting means deciding what changes you should make in the process you've tested if you're going to implement it permanently. And since this is a cycle, you then decide what your next plan is.

The Hospital Executive's Guide to Emergency Department Management

FIGURE 6.3

THE MODEL FOR IMPROVEMENT USING RAPID-CYCLE TESTING

Three
Questions

Testing
Changes

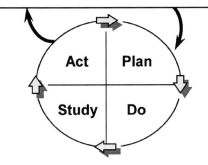

Source: Langley G., Moen R., Nolan K., Nolan T., Norman C., Provost L. *The Improvement Guide.*
San Francisco: Jossey-Bass, 2000. p. 24.

An example of rapid-cycle testing is using x-ray quick reads. Here's how the cycle might unfold. In the first step, which we'll call cycle 1a, we try a pilot—quick reads of x-rays on one shift. As we try it, we monitor the lengths of stay (LOS) for patients with x-rays and the error rate from those quick reads. We review the results with radiology. In cycle 1b, we revise the documentation process and use quick reads on all shifts for two days. In cycle 1c, we redesign the viewing area and continue this trial of quick reads for two weeks. In cycle 1d, we make quick reads standard practice—and continue to monitor results. Figure 6.4 illustrates how using multiple cycles (the quick reads and two others) in this way can lead to specific improvements.

FIGURE 6.4

USING DATA IN RAPID-CYCLE TESTING

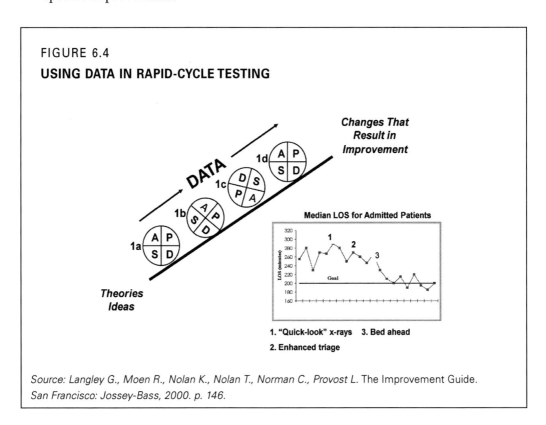

Source: Langley G., Moen R., Nolan K., Nolan T., Norman C., Provost L. *The Improvement Guide.* San Francisco: Jossey-Bass, 2000. p. 146.

The Hospital Executive's Guide to Emergency Department Management

Pointers for the Journey

As you proceed, make sure you collect data. That way, you know whether the change was an improvement and you can tell your story when you succeed. But keep in mind the lesson about gathering too much data. Your written plan and your core team should help you focus on precisely what sorts of data to review. The flip side of too much data is the absence of data during performance improvement subprojects. Not having data and/or metrics for measuring improvement often undercuts improvement efforts. Use a dashboard and communicate what the data are showing you. Keep the data coming regularly. We recommend the use of electronic tracking systems, as long as they are easy to read and use.

Provide incentives to foster healthy competition. These can be financial incentives, promotions, and perks. But make sure everyone on the team knows what the key metrics are for these incentives. You want to build teamwork with competition, not disrupt it. As part of this emphasis, offer plenty of coaching. Determining from the start how often coaching will take place and who will coach helps with this process.

AN EXAMPLE: ESTABLISHING A SUPER TRACK

Let's consider a hypothetical example to show how we might implement a specific subproject in our overall improvement project. We want to develop a super track in our ED. First, we need to decide what measures we're going to use, and we choose the following two:

- Time from patient entry to the ED to being seen by a clinician in the super track

- Time from patient entry to the ED to discharge from the ED

For each measure, we set a corresponding goal:

- Less than 15 minutes and within 30 days

- Less than 60 minutes and within 60 days

Before we start, we describe in writing the current performance of these two measures. Doing so gives us a baseline against which we can gauge progress. Once we start, we monitor data and document progress. These actions will help us as we refine this subproject and plan further subprojects. (Figure 6.5 shows how you can document the process).

FIGURE 6.5

DEVELOPING A SUPER TRACK: ASSESSING PROGRESS

Element	Accomplished and working well	Ideas for improvement	Specific things to do
Profile of patient demand by hour	Yes		
Profile of average service times		Understand Takt time*	Determine Takt time based on potential demand for the super track and determine the current average service time for Level 4 and 5 patients
System for patient segmentation		Sort Level 4 and 5 patients from the emergency severity index triage system	Identify conditions for the super track and historical patterns
Staffing mix		Physician assistant, RN, technician	Discuss staffing with leadership and talk to the staff and solicit interest

*Takt time: the maximum time per unit allowed to produce a product in order to meet demand

Reviews by senior leaders

We emphasized earlier the importance of having senior leaders involved in the project. An article from the Institute for Healthcare Improvement (IHI) points out that a project that produces significant, noticeable results sends a signal throughout the organization, but a project that produces superficial results sends one as well, one that will impede implementation of processes that bring lasting, positive change.[4] For this reason, senior leaders should review the project regularly as it proceeds. In doing so, their purpose is fourfold:

- To ask, "Is the project on track, or is it likely to fail?"

- If it is not achieving the intended results, to ask why.

- To provide guidance, support, and stimulus to the project team.

- To decide whether the project should be stopped.

In regard to the second point, the leaders should determine whether the failure to achieve comes from a:

- Lack of organizational will

- Lack of good ideas

- Failure to execute changes

Leaders should be well prepared for review meetings. The IHI article also emphasizes focusing on how the project aligns with system goals, keeping well informed on progress, and communicating clearly with the project manager before meetings.

During those meetings, the senior leader should clarify the project's aim, ask about measures, review data, encourage positive developments, discuss trends, and if the project falls short of aims, determine what needs to be done to get back on track.

An overall view of implementation

Keep system goals in mind at each stage, including any measures established, standards of performance, and timelines. Set out your plans for the next 90 or 120 days, listing tests and activities, who is responsible for implementing them, and by when. Then break down those periods and tests into shorter intervals and subprojects. Keep in mind intermediate goals as you proceed, including measures, performance standards, and timelines.

The following is a list of critical factors your project must have if it is going to succeed:

- An engaged and informed leadership

- Deployment of adequate resources

- Effective meetings (with the core team meeting at least weekly and the project team meeting every other week or monthly)

- Passionate, effective people

- A culture of improvement

- Finite action plans with clear sequencing and tempo (30, 60, 90, 120 days)

- Sustained execution

CASE STUDY   Taking over a new emergency department

The situation

BestPractices assumed the exclusive services agreement to staff a metropolitan Illinois community-based hospital with a 72,000-annual-visit ED volume in June 2006.

What we did

BestPractices recruited a seasoned medical director and a new associate medical director to lead the team. Over the course of three years, 12 new physicians were recruited to join the new team and the BestPractices management system was fully implemented. Key components of the BestPractices operations management system included:

- Enhanced ED section meetings to serve as a change management forum

- A hospitalwide patient flow symposium and private coaching process

- Performance evaluations, including nursing surveys, that were conducted twice a year on all clinicians

- Press Ganey survey data reported on a clinician-specific basis for all clinicians; quarterly trends demonstrated performance on the four key areas and provided follow-up coaching activity

- Coding in-services and Creating the Risk-Free ED training

- Intranet-based secure clinician performance feedback and training resources

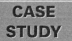

Taking over a new emergency department (cont.)

The results

FIGURE 6.6

PHASE 1 ED RENOVATION RESULTS

Metric	Before	After	Conclusion
Press Ganey Doctor Box mean	81	89	Steady improvement through individual, focused coaching
Patients who left without being seen	1.1%	1.2%	Best in class— no change during transition
Treat-and-release LOS	> 200 min	< 180 min	Modest improvement even through department renovation
Physician productivity	5.0 RVU/hour	6.2 RVU/hour	Pay-for-performance compensation plan was implemented.

Next steps

In September 2009, an advanced triage unit opened in conjunction with the second phase of the ED renovation. The new unit, staffed by a physician, treats less-acute patients and serves as a workup unit for moderately acute patients, thereby diverting patients into the rest of the ED and pushing an efficient patient stream. Initial results exceed expectations, and this unit is poised to fulfill an essential role when the ED enters Phase III of the renovation and has 25% less beds for a 15-month period.

References

1. Shulkin, D. "Why quality improvement efforts in healthcare fail and what can be done about it." *American Journal of Medical Quality.* Volume 15, No. 2, March-April, 2000.

2. Kaplan, H., How Can We Optimize the Success of QI Teams? Institute for Health Care Improvement. Results Collaborative Web-based seminar, 2007.

3. Jensen, K., Mayer, T., Welch, S., Haraden, C. Leadership for Smooth Patient Flow. Chicago: Health Administration Press, 2007.

4. Reinertsen, J., Pugh, M., Nolan, T. Executive Review of Improvement Projects: A Primer for CEOs and other Senior Leaders (PDF). Institute for Healthcare Improvement. Available at: *www.chqi.ca/Resources/Leadership.aspx.*

7

Culture and
Change Management

There is nothing more difficult to carry out ... more doubtful of success,
nor more dangerous to handle than to initiate a new order of things.
—*Machiavelli,* The Prince

When you make major changes in your ED, the key to success is changing the culture. Unfortunately, people fear change. If you're going to change a culture, understanding what culture is before you start can help. Here's one definition of culture:

A shared, learned symbolic system of values, beliefs, and attitudes that
shapes and influences perception and behavior; an abstract "mental blue-
print" or "mental code."[1]

And here's the short version: "It's the way we do things around here."

Keep that short definition in mind, because it explains people's resistance to change. People are used to acting certain ways, carrying out tasks in set processes, and change seems to challenge the validity of those ways. Many improvement vessels have foundered on the sea of custom and inertia.

Resistance can be obvious from the start: The physicians don't support the team and won't participate or there's a lack of leadership guiding the process. However, resistance can also manifest itself less obviously, such as when:

- Agreement is superficial, because there's no follow-through

- Progress is slow

- Apathy permeates the atmosphere

- In lieu of making progress, team members offer excuses

Breaking Free of Gravity

Sociologist Kurt Lewin says achieving organizational change first requires shocking a system out of its inertia.[2] Next, processes need to be adjusted to transform that system. Finally, those new or revised processes must be cemented into the system to create the new culture or "the way we do things now."

Lewin describes the successful change process in terms of driving forces versus restraining forces, using an analogy from physics: The force of a moving object must overcome gravity to keep in motion. In organizational culture change, the moving object is trust. Gravity is inertia. Trust must exceed inertia for the system to change. The most important element in establishing trust is communication.

We can borrow from physics again to show the forces operating when you bring change into an organizational system (Figure 7.1). Driving forces are the improvement processes you are introducing. Restraining forces are the resisting behaviors that develop from a state of inertia when it is challenged. Driving forces must exceed restraining forces for change to occur. In contrast to the way physical nature operates, however, moving productivity higher in organizations requires us to reduce restraining forces, not increase driving forces—an observation that seems counterintuitive to many of us.

FIGURE 7.1

AN ORGANIZATIONAL FORCE FIELD MODEL

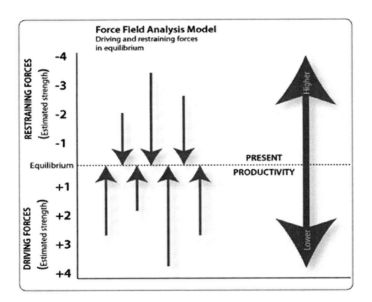

Source: Lewin, K. Resolving Social Conflicts: Selected Papers on Group Dynamics. New York: Harper & Row, 1948.

The notion of restraining and driving forces can help you focus on what you want to achieve and what obstacles are blocking your improvement process. One way to organize yourself initially is by writing down ideas (Figure 7.2). It can help you see what you're up against more clearly.

FIGURE 7.2

CHARTING OPPOSING FORCES

Driving Forces	Restraining Forces

Source: Lewin, K. Resolving Social Conflicts: Selected Papers on Group Dynamics. New York: Harper & Row, 1948.

Lewin also describes the movement of individuals within the process of systematic change. He places them in four "A" stages: beginning with awareness, moving to acceptance, then to adoption, and finally to advocacy. Knowing this pattern is useful as you strive to change your culture.

How to Change a Culture

As you prepare to implement your project, you should start by asking the following questions:

- Does your team's will match your aims?

- Do your resources match your aims?

- Do your ideas match your aims?

- Are you working on the right problems and the right opportunities?

For the last question, rapid-cycle testing (see Figure 6.3) can help determine the answers. You should ask three questions: What are we trying to accomplish? How will we know that the change is an improvement? What changes can we make that will result in an improvement? Then run a small-scale test of the changes, monitor them, and assess the results. For the second question in the bulleted list, be aware that the beginning of a project requires more resources than later stages to enable team building, learning, and initial implementation. It is also important to note that enthusiasm, effort, and resource allocation will fade if the project drags on.

Resistance to change does not necessarily result from a desire to maintain the status quo. Most people have experienced attempts at change that weren't successful and weren't pleasant, and most people have gone through changes that did happen but that weren't for the better. So always keep these guidelines in mind: Change should be smart, specific, measurable, actionable, relevant, and time specific.

Actions to change your culture should proceed from careful planning and should help achieve the goals of a coherent vision.

The following are the strategies to unlock successful culture change:

- Communicate at all times with everyone

- Involve senior leaders

- Develop team leaders

- Create ownership

Communicate, communicate, communicate

Talk with every group you come into contact with in the system and explain what the project is intended to accomplish and give progress reports as you proceed. Point out why the current processes are not working as optimally as they should and how the planned changes will reach system goals. Allow venting but move on quickly to constructive discussion. (See Figure 7.3 for communication strategies to reduce resistance).

To reduce physician resistance, you should answer some questions first. For example, what do you want the physicians to do? What role should individual doctors play—team leader, team player, cheerleader? You should define these roles and communicate your expectations for them. Doctors respond to data, so it is important to share the data you're tracking with them, as well as what the data revealed about existing operations. Physicians want to be compared to their peers, want to earn financial incentives, and favor evidence-based practice. Use this information when communicating goals, expectations, and progress to physicians.

FIGURE 7.3

COMMUNICATION TECHNIQUES FOR OVERCOMING RESISTANCE TO CHANGE

Bring the resistance to the surface:

- "I'd like to hear your thoughts on this."

- "Tell me what concerns you about this."

Show you're listening and empathize:

- "You're right that this will mean some inconvenience."

- "I can understand how that could be a problem for you."

- "Is there anything else that you see as a problem?"

Probe further and explore options:

- "I want to understand your assumptions about this and how it will affect you."

- "How can this be made to work from your point of view?"

Summarize what you have heard:

- "Here's what I've heard you say."

- "Let me review what we've covered."

Source: Block, P. Flawless Consulting, San Francisco: Jossey-Bass, 2000.

Get senior leaders involved

When engaging senior leaders, it is important to understand the organizational goals that motivate leaders. Frame your project to show that it influences those goals. Show how this project complements other key areas that work well in the organization and look for potential allies among senior leaders.

Senior leaders are not the only potential allies. Physicians can also be powerful allies when implementing change in an ED culture. No matter how successful you are in enlisting senior administrative leaders in your project, don't overlook the fact that leaders are not likely to achieve system-level improvement without the enthusiasm, knowledge, cultural clout, and personal leadership of physicians. Get key physician leaders involved early and keep them involved as you proceed. An effective approach is to let them decide what data to monitor and what constitutes appropriate statistical supervision.

Determine who is the key physician thought leader most likely to influence attitudes as you change processes, and involve that physician on the flow committee.

Develop team leaders

In the early stages of the project, you should take advantage of innovators and early adopters and work with them. But don't ignore early resisters, who as the four-A process unfolds can potentially move to awareness—if you communicate effectively—and eventually to advocacy. Everyone has the potential to lead, which we phrase as a principle: All teach, all learn.

The way to implement this principle is to continually coach your staff. Establish stretch goals. Give your team members feedback. Give them the tools to improve through specific coaching and remember to involve them in this process. It is important to let them articulate their perspectives and to listen to them. Kotter's principles for leading change are to plan short-term victories from the start. Then consolidate your gains, make them part of the new order in the ED, and move on.

Project leaders and sponsors should stay in touch with the improvement efforts, visiting the team often, and ensuring that the team has the resources and support it needs. Leaders should give regular updates on progress to the team and issue reminders of what needs to be done regularly.

Most obstacles that improvement projects face involve management of people. Accordingly, managing people effectively solves most problems. Developing leaders on your team is an essential step to moving past barriers.

Owning Part of the Team

Businesses often reward employees—top management on down the line—with stock in the company. This practice takes advantage of psychology; people will naturally work harder at a task if they feel invested in the results. We defined culture as a "shared system of values." Many organizations lack a strong sense of values. Strong cultures are high minded, with a set of values the people within them believe in and are willing to work for.

People care about what they do.

Most workers in EDs care about providing high-quality service to their patients. If your improvement project leads to changes that enhance your team members' ability to provide such care, it is likely to spark enthusiasm for the changes among them. If you focus on a few important values, you can change the culture.

Psychologist Abraham Maslow developed a pyramid-shaped hierarchy of needs, with physiological needs such as dietary and safety needs at the base levels of the pyramid[3]. As you travel up the pyramid, social needs become more important, including a sense of belonging. Self-esteem is higher up, and at the top is self-actualization. So in addition to financial incentives, your team members are likely to be motivated by being part of a culture with values they share and are passionate about. If you can clearly convey that the changes your ED is making align with the strong values your team holds regarding high-quality care, then you will help propel your team toward change. Changing the culture then becomes considerably less formidable.

People seldom object to changes that they initiate. When they feel forced or manipulated into changing, however, they often react by resisting. So besides showing how the changes will enhance shared values, you should emphasize enlightened self-interest. Help your team members answer this question: What's in it for me? The answer is not simply financial incentive, although that's part of it. Working in an effective ED that patients want to come to, one recognized for high-quality care and customer service, creates a more pleasant environment to work in. Your staff members will value that environment out of self-interest as much as finding fulfillment in shared values. Who wouldn't want to work in a pleasant, smoothly operating workplace?

Envisioning the Future

Aside from constant communication, it is equally important to create a vision of what the changed culture will look like. Leaders should help doctors, nurses, and other staff members on the team envision the same picture. It will help motivate the team from within and bring the changed culture about. Three of Kotter's eight principles for leading change have to do with the vision of change. Kotter points out that failure to successfully embrace those principles are common reasons for failed attempts to change organizational culture. Specifically in regard to vision, those failures take the form of:

- Underestimating the power of vision

- Undercommunicating the vision

- Permitting obstacles to block the vision

To convince staff members to embrace the vision, you must create a sense of urgency. Most change programs fail at the outset because their leaders fail to properly communicate the urgency of the circumstances requiring a change in culture. If you want to succeed, more than 75% of the staff members in the ED must believe that business as usual is unacceptable.

Develop a compelling vision for a better of way of doing things; focus on quality, patient safety, service, and improved working conditions for the healthcare staff. Emphasize improving quality and service, as well as professional pride. When communicating your vision, the following points are key:

- **Repetition:** Communicate your message frequently

- **Consistency:** Convey the same message every time

- **Accuracy:** Do not tell your team lies, half-truths, or sugar-coated pabulum

Psychologist Albert Bandura's social cognitive theory says people who are motivated to change believe that the outcome of the change is important; they view any proposed changes as connected to the envisioned outcome, and they are confident they can make the proposed changes. Communication throughout the process, coaching, and feedback all relate significantly to these motivators.

Cementing the Changes

When you start changing your culture, you need some short-term successes. So start small and build up, making sure you celebrate those successes and credit those involved in them publicly and personally through feedback. (Figure 7.4 offers a useful approach, both for setting up some quick victories and developing a strategy for longer-term challenges). Assessing the impact of changes helps keep your strategy connected to the envisioned outcome. Again, get it in writing!

FIGURE 7.4

ACTION PLANS FOR THE CHANGE PROCESS

	EASY	HARD
High Impact		
Low Impact		

Once you've reached some of your more easily attainable goals, raise the bar higher and set new goals. Make sure the goals are connected to the outcome and are clearly understood by your team. It is also imperative to establish the changed processes that enabled you to successfully meet your goal as the processes that should be followed from this point on—this is the way we do things now.

When consolidating your gains, make sure you keep communicating. Publicize your successes and provide frequent status updates. Review completed actions and assess what you've learned—what worked well, what could be improved, and what lessons can be applied to future actions. Monitor your processes and measure and track data. Transfer responsibility for operations to ongoing management from the project team.

Keep following this procedure, and you'll be on your way to changing the culture in your ED.

References

1. Dahl, K. *Culture*. 2001. Retrieved October 10, 2007, from the Eastern Oregon University website: *http://www2.eou.edu/~kdahl/cultdef.html.*

2. Lewin, K. *Resolving Social Conflicts: Selected Papers on Group Dynamics.* New York: Harper & Row, 1948.

3. Maslow, A. *Toward a Psychology of Being.* Third Edition. New York: Wiley & Sons, 1968, 1999.

Patient Safety and Risk Reduction

In 2001, the Institute of Medicine published the report *To Err Is Human: Building a Safer Healthcare System,* which caught the attention of the public. It concluded that between 44,000 and 98,000 deaths occurred each year in the United States as a result of adverse events to patients. Just using the lower number of 44,000 meant that adverse events constituted the seventh leading cause of deaths in the nation, exceeding deaths due to motor-vehicle accidents, breast cancer, and AIDS. The Dynamics Research Corporation (DRC) studied error rates in EDs and identified an average of nine teamwork errors per case. The DRC study found that 50% of the harm that occurred because of errors could have been prevented.

The human cost of this error rate is obvious. But there are other costs to hospital systems, as well. Emergency-medicine group practices spend between 5% and 10% of their cost of services on medical-malpractice premiums, which represents the third largest expense category behind personnel and coding/billing. Proactively managing risk and achieving higher standards of patient safety clearly benefits patients, emergency-medicine groups, and hospital systems, through improved quality, service, and finances.

Perfection Vs. Improvement

Only the mediocre are at their best all the time.

—Oscar Wilde

More than two thousand years ago, Hippocrates issued his primary guideline for physicians: "First, do no harm." He did not say: "Make no mistakes." Expectations of healthcare workers throughout the ages have not included perfection. In the past, peer-review and quality-assurance programs operated under two guiding assumptions:

- Increased physician vigilance leads to flawless performance

- A few physicians can be identified as the principal source of errors

Those assumptions are unrealistic. Highly motivated, skilled, and dedicated professionals can, do, and will make errors. And a study by Glauber et al. (2000) found that errors were evenly distributed among 13 of 18 ED physicians in their sample. Errors are going to happen. But accepting that fact does not mean you cannot reduce the number of errors, and more importantly, prevent harm to your patients.

FIGURE 8.1

PROBABILITY OF PERFORMING PERFECTLY BY NUMBER OF ELEMENTS AT INCREASING SUCCESS RATES

Number of elements	Probability at 95% rate	Probability at 99% rate	Probability at 99.9% rate	Probability at 99.99% rate
1	95.0%	99.0%	99.9%	99.99%
25	28.0%	78.0%	98.0%	99.8%
50	8.0%	61.0%	95.0%	99.5%
100	0.6%	37.0%	90.0%	99.0%

The vertical axis of Figure 8.1 shows an increasing number of elements, such as the number of patients or the number of decisions made during each patient encounter. Going through the rows of the table gives you the probability of error-free performance for a specified number of elements per overall success rate. For example, in an ED that sees 100 patients per day, each with one decision, if the probability of treating one patient without error for that particular facility is 95%, then the probability of treating all 100 patients without error is less than 1%. That statistic should humble us.

But when you increase your success rate for one element from 95% to 99.9%, the probability for treating 100 patients without error is 90%. That statistic should encourage us. Reducing your rate of errors can pay dramatic dividends.

Living with 99.9% success?

A success rate of 99.9% sounds exceedingly good—in school that rate would net us an A+ and plenty of scholarship offers. But succeeding 99.9% of the time also means:

- 84 unsafe airline landings each day

- One major plane crash every three days

- 16,000 items of lost mail every hour

- 37,000 ATM errors per hour

Boosting the success rate in your ED from 99.9% to 99.99% can have important ramifications for your patients.

A culture of safety and preventing harm

As healthcare professionals, we want to provide high-quality, reliable service. Organizations that achieve high quality consistently are not only concerned with how well they are doing; they are also concerned with what can potentially go wrong. They focus continually on what can go wrong and how to fix or prevent it. Still, errors occur every day in our EDs. Organizations should accept this fact and find ways to reduce the frequency of errors and, perhaps more importantly, prevent harm when errors do occur. The following are five principles of reliability and safety:

- All people make mistakes

- "First, do no harm" does not mean do not make any mistakes

- Most error-prone or high-risk situations are predictable, manageable, and preventable

- A strong culture of safety is essential

- A collaborative approach results in better outcomes, and an organization's preoccupation with failure is essential

A culture of safety focuses on reducing errors, predicting what may go wrong, learning from errors that do happen, and preventing harm when errors occur. A culture of safety makes errors visible when they do occur, mitigates their impact, and doesn't play the blame game. The old peer-review and quality-assurance models stressed who was at fault, but the new collaborative models clearly convey that the leadership understands staff members do not come to work to make errors and the organization—as a whole—wants to minimize the risk.

A Systematic Approach

Many people throughout your organization make errors, not just a few who stand out. You should emphasize systems rather than individuals. In an article on errors in medicine in 1994, Lucian Leape noted that the 1979 accident at the Three Mile Island nuclear power plant in Pennsylvania caused psychologists and human-factors engineers to reexamine their theories about human error. Many of the errors that led to the incident were caused by faulty interface design, others by complex interactions and breakdowns that neither operators nor their instruments could detect. Subsequent disasters in the 1980s, notably the Bhopal chemical explosion in India and the nuclear accident at Chernobyl in the Soviet Union, demonstrated that operator errors were only part of the explanation of failures in complex systems. Disasters of this magnitude resulted from a series of major failures due to organization design that occurred long before the accident—failures that caused operator errors and made them impossible to reverse.

Errors are an intrinsic performance characteristic of complex systems.

Faulty processes typically account for 85% of problems in a system, and human inadequacy accounts for only 15%. Hospital systems are no different. Charles Vincent and his colleagues pioneered the use of an investigative process for medical accidents in which hospital staff members comprehensively examine all factors that could be involved. They reported in 2000 that this process uncovers multiple system defects and reveals that accidents result from multiple causes of which the obvious human error is often the least important. Robust systems anticipate common cognitive errors and build in safeguards to identify and counteract them before they affect vital processes.

Adverse events, near misses, and errors waiting to happen are opportunities to learn about the system—near misses reveal weaknesses in the system just as effectively as errors but at a much lower cost in human misery and wasted resources. After an error or near miss occurs, organizations should ask the following two questions:

- Why would this mistake happen?

- What redesign would make it less likely?

Examining human performance has the potential to help organizations continually improve their systems and reduce bad outcomes due to errors. T. W. Nolan (2000) describes three ways to increase the safety and reliability of a medical system:

- Design the system to prevent errors

- Design procedures to make errors visible when they do occur so they can be intercepted

- Design procedures for mitigating the adverse effects of errors when they are not detected and intercepted

Nolan suggests several actions to achieve these goals: reduce complexity, optimize information processing, automate wisely, use constraints, and mitigate unwanted side effects of change. If errors are an inescapable part of complex systems, the more you can simplify processes and the more steps you can eliminate, the more likely you will be able to cut down the number of potential errors in the system.

For example, Espinosa and Nolan examined a project to reduce errors emergency physicians make in interpreting radiographs and the impact of that reduction on quality and patient safety:

The emergency department redesigned the process of X-ray interpretation to include the emergency physician's initial interpretation, the radiologist's follow-up interpretation within 12 hours as a quality-control measure, and a recall procedure when a team member noticed a clinically significant error. The redesign reduced four processes for interpreting the radiograph to one.

As a result of the changes, the false negative rate fell from 3% to 0.3%, the time from ordering plain film to their return to the ED decreased by 50%, and the time from patients' arrival in the ED with trauma to an extremity to discharge dropped by 50%. Patient satisfaction rose from the 18th percentile to above the 95th percentile.

Reducing Errors and Preventing Harm

The following are important principles to keep in mind when redesigning your processes and establishing a culture of safety in your ED:

- Hire the right team

- Emphasize teamwork and communication

- Implement after-action reviews

- Emphasize error reporting

- Manage high-risk presentations

- Conduct patient-safety rounds

- Cultivate patient satisfaction

- Relentlessly focus on operations

- Build reliability into your system

MILITARY AVIATION AND EMERGENCY MEDICINE: THE TEAMWORK CONNECTION

For the aviation industry establishing a culture of safety is vital and, subsequently, has been an area of focus for a long time. Many safety techniques that other industries have adopted come from aviation. Military aviation, in particular, has a significant connection to emergency medicine. Studies of crashes and near mishaps in the military revealed that the single biggest cause of accidents was miscommunication. In response, the military developed crew resource management (CRM), a training method that focuses on teaching teammates to work together as a coordinated unit and to communicate effectively. This kind of training greatly reduced the number of accidents.

DRC, which was involved in the military development of CRM, and other organizations later adopted the principles of CRM and implemented them in emergency medicine. DRC's MedTeams program is one approach. Even though hospitals using MedTeams have significantly improved the quality of care in EDs, a primary motivation behind the program has always been enhancing patient safety. You can teach teamwork skills and situational awareness—both of which are valuable in establishing a culture of safety. A technique that helps reinforce situational awareness is SBAR: situation, background, assessment, and recommendation. Team members use it when communicating with each other regarding a patient. The following are a description of each SBAR component

Situation: Describe the situation with clear facts and figures (pulse rate, respiration, and concerns).
Background: Describe the patient's background.
Assessment: Give a clear assessment of the problem.
Recommendations: Make recommendations on managing the case.

This procedure may seem simple, but having an established protocol of this sort helps your team members communicate effectively and succinctly in your ED. Similar to military aviation, clear communication and coordinated teamwork implement a culture of safety.

Looking back after the dust settles

Studies of errors across various industries have shown that the initial blame for 70% to 80% of errors falls on the last person involved in the situation. However, subsequent investigation of the event usually reveals that the last person involved accounts for less than 20% of the error. Conducting after-action reviews provides a method to examine what went wrong in the system when a mistake occurs.

When reviewing the cause of accidents, organizations should focus less on the individual who makes the error and more on preexisting organizational factors because of the complex chain of events that can lead to an adverse outcome (Vincent et al. 2000). The ultimate cause, for example, may be excessive workload and training deficiencies.

During an after-action review, you should ask these questions:

- What were our intended results and how were we going to measure them?

- What challenges could we have anticipated in this case?

- What have we or others learned from experiencing similar situations?

- What will enable us to succeed in a similar case?

You should also talk with all of the key people involved. You can learn sequentially about the case through multiple discussions and fine-tune your follow-up questions based on previous conversations. After you talk to everyone involved, you should go back and talk to the first people interviewed again—this time armed with your acquired knowledge about the events surrounding the case.

Catching the errors

If the old models emphasized who was at fault, the underlying atmosphere they created was fear. Punishment drives errors underground where they are not reported and no one can learn from them. This environment leaves the system unchanged, and the errors will continue to occur.

Fear never makes for good policy or good practice.

In order to learn from errors and near misses and establish a safer, more effective department, you must take a fundamentally different approach to errors by establishing a nonpunitive approach. Your staff members must believe reporting errors will not get them in trouble, and they must believe reporting errors is a top priority of your operation.

An error-report chart is one way to encourage team members to report near misses and mistakes (see Figure 8.2 for an example). It should be simple to create and follow. It provides an effective way to learn what is happening in your ED. You should use it for three months and track the categories. At the end of three months, examine the patterns, and make process improvements.

FIGURE 8.2

AN ERROR-REPORT CHART

Incident	Record Number	Type	Suggestions for Improvement	Results

---

Reducing and managing risk

Flow principles can also help you to manage high-risk situations and reduce the risk. If you know who's going to come to your ED and why they're coming, then you can prepare to handle high-risk situations. Examine the top 10 to 20 closed malpractice cases with the greatest prevalence for emergency physicians and establish best practices for treating these types of cases. The following list represents the top ten.

1. Acute myocardial infarction

2. Appendicitis

3. Meningitis

4. Chest pain

5. Open wounds

   The Hospital Executive's Guide to Emergency Department Management

6. Abdominal/pelvic pain

7. Pneumonia

8. Spinal fracture

9. Aortic aneurysm

10. Male genitalia

For example, the best practice for every patient with an acute onset of testicular pain and a clinical finding of testicular torsion includes the following steps:

- An immediate call to the urologist

- Attempted manual detorsion

- Immediate surgery as definitive treatment

Every patient with testicular torsion as a presumptive diagnosis should receive an ultrasound and a urological consultation. Making this procedure standard practice enables you to clinically diagnose testicular torsion definitively. If the procedure is embedded into your ED practice, the emergency physicians know it, the nurses know it, and the attending physicians know it.

Following this approach enabled our EDs to reduce misdiagnosing testicular torsion by 70% in one year, which resulted in a decrease in malpractice-insurance premiums. In addition, satisfaction rates increased among physicians, nurses, and patients.

Using an evidence-based format to standardize treatment for the other closed-case malpractice experiences enables you to manage risk in these situations effectively and reduce risk significantly.

Taking a walk around the ED

Clinical and administrative leaders should conduct regular safety rounds throughout the department to see for themselves how operations are proceeding, how the ED looks, and to speak with staff members and patients so that they can learn what areas to focus on for improvement. Is the department clean? Is it working effectively? Is it clinically safe?

The Institute for Healthcare Improvement has an initiative known as WalkRounds—developed by Allan Frankel and colleagues (2003)—that provides a detailed process for conducting rounds. The process enables senior leaders and various staff members to discuss safety conditions in the department confidentially. The following are examples of routine questions that leaders should ask to elicit information:

- Can you think of any events in the past day that have resulted in prolonged stays for a patient?

- Have there been any near misses?

- Have there been any incidents recently that concern you or your team members?

- What can we do to prevent an adverse event?

When you have established a blame-free culture of error reporting, these conversations can provide leaders with valuable intelligence from the people doing the work on the ED floor. These rounds help you identify weaknesses and give you opportunities to improve.

Don't forget to enter information gathered in these rounds into a tracking database, categorized by contributing factors. Tracking and analyzing data helps you respond effectively to safety issues.

Keeping the patients satisfied

Patient satisfaction and patient safety go hand in hand; when patients are satisfied, usually conditions are safer. A clean department, for example, is a safer one.

As in many other aspects of ED operations, effective communication leads to more satisfied patients. For example, 71% of patients who sued for malpractice cited a poor relationship with staff as the reason for their legal action. Of those patients, 32% felt deserted and 29% felt devalued. Good communication not only reduces the risk of malpractice litigation, but also inherently makes the ED safer.

How your ED handles complaints should be as important as preventing them. The hospital's patient advocate staff should be involved in receiving complaints and serving as an unbiased representative of the patients. The ED's medical director should follow a protocol for resolving patient complaints with timely and detailed personal contact with the patient involved. Take advantage of the opportunity to gather data you can track and analyze for trends. Circulate the results of this analysis with all clinicians in the department to improve performance.

Stay focused on ongoing operations

The pessimist complains about the wind. The optimist expects it to change.
The realist adjusts the sails.

—William Arthur Ward

Following the principles we discussed on improving flow will help you improve safety as well as efficiency. When you're tracking data, monitoring a dashboard, testing changes, and performing the other techniques of smoothing flow, you'll also be reducing complexity, improving coordination and communication, and decreasing the likelihood of error. A culture of safety is obsessed with failure. The more you can monitor operations, examine what is happening, and adjust the processes, the more mistakes you can prevent. Coaching is an important part of operations. To reduce risk, organize diagnostic categories for high-risk conditions. Provide education on common approaches to these conditions to physicians, mid-level providers, and nurses. Use white papers and PowerPoint® presentations to outline evaluation, diagnosis, and treatment for each category. Then follow up with competency quizzes to test how well your team has absorbed the educational material. You want to increase both competency and accountability.

Educational programs should have a pediatrics component in addition to an adult component, and you should ensure one component focuses specifically on nursing. The adult and nursing modules should address the 10 conditions listed earlier in the section on managing risk. The pediatric module should include these categories:

- Pediatric meningitis

- Asthma

- Neonatal evaluation

- Abdominal pain

- Shock

- Child abuse

- Hip pain

- Vomiting

New clinicians should be required to complete these modules within a prescribed time—we recommend 90 days. Some group practices require annual or biannual recertification to be eligible for certain bonuses. This process heightens participation on a team, creates a common language for clinicians and nursing staff, and supports a learning environment to enable your staff to better understand certain clinical cases and enables them to intervene in a comprehensive and predictable manner. The more you simplify decision-making, the more you increase effectiveness and reduce risk.

Make the system reliable

Reliability comes from emphasizing several factors:

- Standardizing processes

- Introducing redundancy

- Identifying critical failures

- Redesigning processes

When you used an automated teller machine (ATM), for example, you used to put in your card and it gave you your money. Then you pushed a button to get your card back. However, people kept forgetting to retrieve their cards. Finally, banks examined the process and redesigned it. With newer ATMs, you must take your card back before the machine dispenses your cash. The redesign built safety and reliability into the ATM system.

We can apply similar principles in medicine. Here's an example dealing with community-acquired pneumonia.

The triage process in an ED is intent on building reliability, so it establishes triggers when someone over 50 years of age arrives with a productive cough, high temperature, and other symptoms suggestive of pneumonia. Triage staff automatically flags that patient for a chest x-ray. Once the physician or midlevel provider makes a diagnosis of pneumonia, another trigger alerts the pharmacy, which then automatically sends a message back to the ED: "Is this patient on the pneumonia pathway?" If the x-ray indicates pneumonia, the radiology department has a trigger in its system that flags pneumonia for the ED and then asks if the patient is being treated accordingly (see Figure 8.3).

FIGURE 8.3

CAP PROTOCOL MODEL

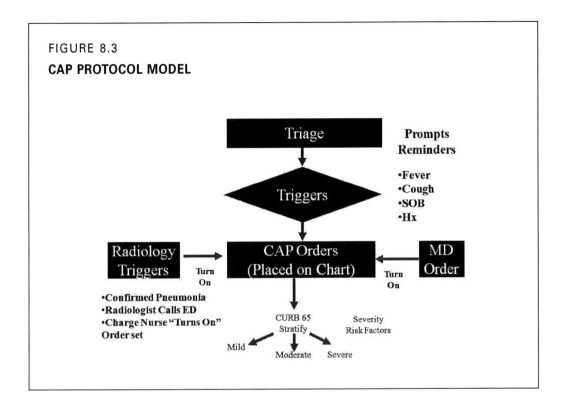

Organizations should standardize information, reporting forms, and procedures to reduce variation. If the layout of your department separates work groups or disrupts processes, then redesign it to smooth actual physical flow within it. Group types of work with similar requirements, and automate repetitive operations.

Building reliability into your system will enable you to go from one error in every 10 cases to one error in every 100. When you achieve that goal, you will have greatly improved the quality of your care and the safety of your environment.

The Role and Necessity of the Dashboard

Consider a typical day. We start our day at a specific time that is usually announced by an alarm, after which we may listen to radio newscasts or TV news reports. We then may pick up a newspaper to review things like the Dow Jones Industrial closing from the prior day and trends on futures, mortgage interest rates, the treasury, etc. We may also get absorbed in sports scores that dissect players' statistics, game statistics, season averages, and trends that seemingly go back to the early 1900s if not before. We may then get our kids off to school and think about things such as their class rank or their GPA. If they're college age or nearing the end of their high school experience, we're thinking about how they're scoring on their SATs or their ACTs.

We then get into our car and think about how many miles per gallon our car gets and what current gas prices are. Throughout the day, we are performing work based on some notion of what our productivity for a given day should be. Before the day is over, we're picking up a gallon of milk and a loaf of bread and contemplating where to get the best buy on a gallon of milk and what the current market average for a loaf of bread is. By the end of the day, we have formally and informally planned and executed many aspects of our daily life based on comparative data or benchmarks. We do this as a means of assessing and evaluating our current performance: What is it now and how does it compare historically or against some competitive benchmark or industry average? We're competitive and we're hired to drive our organizations to achieve excellence, not mediocrity.

How well do you know the performance of your ED? How well do the people managing and filling roles in your ED understand their performance? Is your ED excellent? Why not? What needs to occur to make it excellent?

Managing an ED without a dashboard is like driving down a major interstate at midnight without headlights. You're on a busy interstate, at night, traveling at high speed with other cars zipping past you. You reach up and turn your headlights off. Can you imagine how that would feel? The analogy is both visceral and real. In the many consulting engagements we perform, we routinely recommend a better grounding, understanding, and use of metrics. It's like turning on the headlights on a dark night.

Where to Start

Organizations should start at a macro level. Collect volume statistics so that there's a thorough understanding of the number of registrations and which visits result in billable encounters. In order to understand which registrations become billable encounters, there must be a reliable means of identifying the registrations that are nonbillable. Within the nonbillable category, there are registrations that are missed revenue opportunities (patients who left without being seen, left without treatment, and left against medical advice). The other nonbillable registrations, which are not a professional-service revenue opportunity, include patients seen by a private attending, direct admissions, patients screened as a result of a sexual assault, wound and suture recheck or removal, other contractual public health visits, etc. Most ED professional groups will bill 90%–95% of department registrations. The other 5%–10% will be registrations that do not result in a billable encounter. It's very important to understand, track, monitor, and manage the non-billable registrations to keep them as low as contractually and reasonably possible.

In addition to the visits, it's important from a macro level to understand the number of ED visit admissions, transfers, and hours the ED is on diversion. The number of hours spent boarding patients awaiting an inpatient bed should be calculated by counting boarding hours at the conclusion of the period from the time a decision to admit has been made until a patient has waited two hours in the ED for an inpatient bed. These statistics should be gathered in a reliable fashion, well understood by the management team, and reviewed routinely at regular intervals (at least monthly). These data should also be analyzed across months and years in order to understand seasonal fluctuations and growth or recession trends in any of these key areas (admissions, transfers, hours on diversion, etc.).

The next category for metrics falls under the general auspices of throughput times. Total length of stay in minutes should be further detailed into patients treated and released and patients treated and admitted. The other throughput time segments that should be captured are:

- Door to triage

- Door to bed

- Door to doctor

- Bed to doctor

- Doctor to departure

- Disposition to departure

For treated and admitted patients, admission decision to bed assignment and bed assignment to departure from ED are very important time segments to monitor. These data will be gleaned from a tracking board and/or the time stamps included in the medical record. This will help reveal the extent to which the ED is effectively preparing the admitted patient and the opportunity for improving the time segment between the decision to admit and the department departure.

You should also look at primary ancillary testing. The radiology turnaround time for plain films, CTs, and ultrasounds should be reviewed monthly, as well as lab turnaround times for, at a minimum, complete blood counts, complete metabolic profiles, urinalyses, and troponins. The primary quality data sets that should be reviewed on a dashboard include core measure data as defined by the Centers for Medicare & Medicaid Services and include:

- Acute STEMI

  - Aspirin on arrival

  - Beta-blocker on arrival

  - Average time from door to thrombolytic drug administration

  - Percent of visits taking less than 30 minutes

  - Average time from door to percutaneous coronary intervention

  - Percent of visits taking less than 90 minutes

- Community-acquired pneumonia testing

  - Percent of patients with oxygen assessment within 24 hours of arrival

  - Percent of blood cultures drawn prior to antibiotics

  - Percent of initial antibiotics consistent with current recommendations

  - Average time from door to antibiotic administration

  - Percent of patients receiving antibiotics within four hours of arrival

The next major area on the dashboard addresses patient-satisfaction survey results.

Depending on which company performs patient-satisfaction survey analysis for your organization, the results should be reviewed either monthly or quarterly. Peer group percentile ranks should be targeted and monitored. Lastly, the dashboard should include specific progress on process improvement projects the department is undertaking.

Creating a useful dashboard is certainly essential; however, the following are challenges you should be aware of and address at the onset.

- **Validate data sources.** You will have multiple data sources identifying the number of emergency visits rendered in a given month, and frequently, each data source will produce a different tally. This is common due to a variety of factors; however, for your dashboard it is imperative that you select one data source that all parties using these data can agree reliably represents the metric being reviewed.

- **Define data sources and qualify limitations of the data source.** This is particularly important in understanding billable versus nonbillable registrations. Involve all shareholders in data reviews and encourage challenging data. Once limitations are understood and documented, however, the data source challenges should cease, unless, of course, a better source is offered for consideration.

- **Publish data in routine and predictable cycles.** This can be monthly, quarterly, or annually—consistency is key. It should be accessible to medical leaders and staff. Many organizations choose to publish certain ED metrics like average wait time on their websites, as well.

 The Hospital Executive's Guide to Emergency Department Management

- **Present data in a hierarchical form.** This way, trended information can more easily guide the reviewer to relevant conclusions. It is also important to have detailed data available for "drill downs" into the data and data audits.

Clinician Dashboard Metrics

The clinician needs individualized metrics in order to understand his or her performance as compared to group peers as well as industry averages. Most of these data are already captured by the coding and billing personnel. Dashboard metrics should consistently reflect the same time periods as metrics supplied to the physicians. For example, if visit data are batched and relative value units (RVU) are summarized by batch days rather than calendar date of service, inconsistencies can result in time worked versus RVUs produced. These nuances within the dashboard presentation should be documented and footnoted so that anyone reviewing the dashboard can readily understand the metrics and definitions and make reasonable conclusions or analyses.

The key metrics the doctors should be aware of relate to their patient velocity (number of patients seen per clinical hour), average length of stay (average number of minutes for patients treated by the physician), and RVUs per hour (this is an index of productivity indicating the number of relative value units produced per clinical hour by the clinician). Additionally, if the patient-satisfaction surveying instrument provides clinician-specific results reporting, this should be routinely distributed to the individual clinician to gain greater insight into feedback from patients he or she treated. (*Note:* It's important to summarize these results over a long enough period of time in order to capture a large enough sample to infer meaning from the survey results.)

With macro metrics, you can provide the clinician driving down the highway without lights a compass heading, general highway speed, and low beams, and with micro metrics, or clinician-specific metrics, you can provide a tachometer, GPS, fuel gauge, tire pressure gauge, etc. The more clinicians are equipped to evaluate their own performance by comparing it to peers, the better they will be able to adjust and improve their performance.

Summary

The old adage goes that if you don't choose a target, you're only assured of never hitting it. Likewise, if goals are not selected and owned in the ED, they're very unlikely to be achieved. Before goals can meaningfully be accepted, the entire ED team must be knowledgeable of current operating metrics. They must have confidence in the metrics being presented to them, and they must have confidence in initiatives that will enable them to make improvements along the path toward goal achievement. This process should be transparent, involve as many of the stakeholders as possible, and become a routine part of how the ED team conducts itself. Metrics should not be used as a hammer to point out inadequacies, but should rather be a benchmark on the road to improvement.

CASE STUDY

Using the ED dashboard as a coaching tool

The situation

- A physician was having performance issues and patient complaints

- The physician had been at the hospital for about one year

- Staff morale was low

The background

The physician had spent one year seeing patients at a 60,000-annual-visit hospital's ED in northern Virginia. While his outcomes were fine, other performance metrics were suffering. His patient velocity was lower than his peers', length-of-stay (LOS) times were higher than his peers', and patients were complaining and dissatisfied. Additionally, coworkers commented that the physician had difficulty relating to others and did not receive feedback well.

BestPractices uses a tool called the 4S Dashboard to track various performance metrics over time, including patient satisfaction, patient velocity, LOS, downcodes, and other indicators. These measures were used to help coach the physician to improve productivity.

What we did

We collated performance numbers for the past year (relative value units, patient velocity, LOS, down-codes, hours worked, and patient satisfaction) from the dashboard and created a series of graphs to show progress over the year (see Figure 9.1).

CASE STUDY

Using the ED dashboard as a coaching tool (cont.)

FIGURE 9.1

SUMMARY SUSTAINABILITY METRICS, 2009

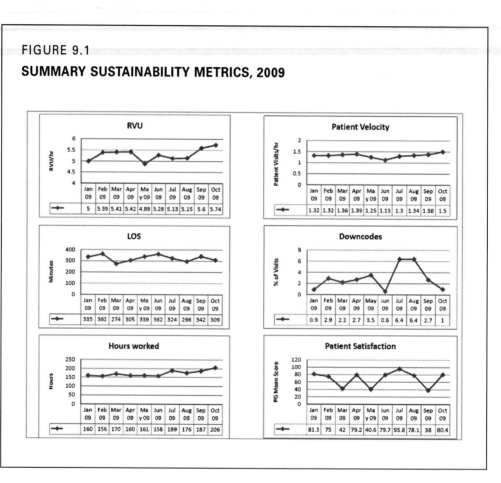

Trended graphs of the physician's performance were compared to the group average over the year. These were then used to create a performance improvement plan with real goals and strategies to help the physician not only become more productive but also to relate better to coworkers and improve his own job satisfaction.

CASE
STUDY

Using the ED dashboard as a coaching tool (cont.)

FIGURE 9.2

PHYSICIAN VERSUS GROUP PERFORMANCE

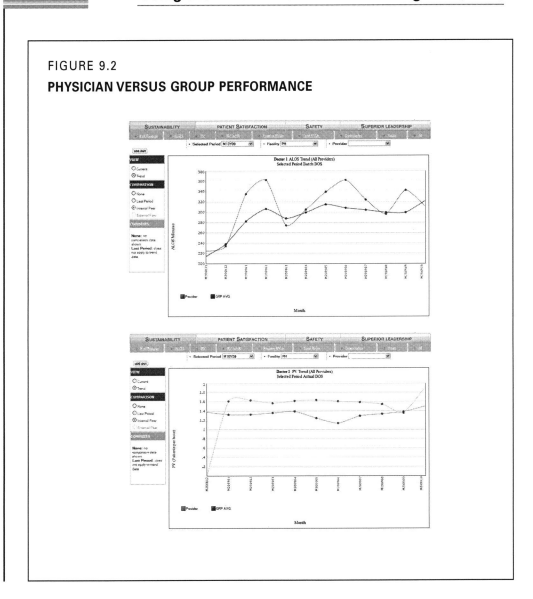

CASE STUDY

Using the ED dashboard as a coaching tool (cont.)

The results

Clearly defined objectives presented and explained by the medical director and operations director helped establish the baseline for this physician. A four-pronged approach was utilized:

- Monthly reports trending results were reviewed and distributed by the medical director and the operations director

- A senior physician mentor was assigned to meet with the younger physician in a consultative/advisory capacity

- Monthly check-ins were scheduled to discuss what was working and what else could be improved

- The physician participated in individual patient-satisfaction coaching and shadowing

Physician Compensation: Productivity-Based Systems

The adage is true: Once you've developed a productivity-based compensation system that works for one group, you've developed a productivity-based compensation system that works for one group. There are certainly tenets and concepts that are transferable; however, what's more important is how the process of moving from the current compensation system to a productivity-based compensation system is forged. This can be particularly important depending on the complexion of the physician group—especially the physician leadership (both formal and informal) within the group.

CHALLENGING CONVERSION

Consider this example of a consulting engagement with a group that was changing from an hourly payment scheme to a productivity-based relative value unit (RVU) compensation system. The planning process went on for several months, and the following are some of the interesting dynamics that characterized the process:

- The practice owner decided not to involve the other doctors in the planning process

- Planning time was minimized in order to roll out the new compensation plan to coincide with the beginning of a calendar year

- The practice owner was totally focused on a belief that there was only one correct way to form this new plan and make the transition from old to new

The transition occurred, even though it had a rocky start that was characterized by a lot of distrust, and it took time to heal the emotional and business wounds that the process left behind. The following is Dan's description of a follow-up conversation some five years after the compensation plan conversion:

"We were 25 miles off the southwest coast of Florida by Marco Island and were experiencing 6-ft. swells. We were in a 25-ft. outboard, and I noticed that the captain was exceedingly adept at being able to anchor the boat so that we rode the swells, didn't put undue tension on the anchor line, and were successfully positioned to enable four of us to fish without getting entangled. I asked the captain his secret, to which he responded, 'You always have to find the sweet spot. The sweet spot exists in that place where the waves pushing the boat toward shore get neutralized by the tide pulling the boat out.' I summarized this story and asked the practice owner if he had it to do over would he have pursued the transition from the old compensation plan to the new compensation plan in a different manner, and did he think he found the sweet spot, balancing pushes and pulls? He noted that he would never make the plan switch the way he had previously and he confessed that he pushed his group needlessly into total distrust and they pulled him through pure hell."

Role in the ED

What is the role of a productivity-based compensation system in your ED? Do you know the characteristics of the current compensation system your emergency professional group uses? Are the right incentives included in the exclusive service agreement between your organization and the emergency physician group and are they fully aligned? Is there enough money at risk to align behavior change to create the right potential for expected outcomes?

It's not uncommon for hospital administrators to answer the previous questions with, "I think so" or "Probably" or, perhaps more honestly, "I sure hope so."

Many nonprofit hospital administrators have been directed by their boards to forge at-risk relationships with physician groups. Although well intentioned, they frequently fall short for several reasons—namely, suspect data collection and reporting, insufficient money at risk, and poorly articulated expectations of all participants in the relationship. Although I am a staunch proponent of hospitals including performance expectations in exclusive service agreements, it has also been my experience that many hospitals fail to have a firm grasp on their current operating metrics and, consequently, have a difficult time keeping track of quantitative measures that demonstrate whether objectives are being met. Although there is clearly room to include performance objectives in exclusive service agreements and tie money to them, it is probably more practical to support your emergency services professional group to implement a productivity-based compensation system as a means of aligning shared goals.

In order to prepare for a productivity-based compensation system, there needs to be a transparent due-diligence process performed on the chart documentation capture and billing processes. If the hospital is involved in coding and billing for the physician group, this due diligence should be transparent and probably performed with the involvement of one or more representatives of the physician group. At any rate, the components that need to be evaluated and either confirmed to be at a level of 99% accuracy or reconfigured to achieve a 99% accuracy rate include the following.

- All patients registered as emergency patients are not billable by the professional service group (nonbillable patients include direct admissions, patients seen by their private attending, rechecks on wound and suture removals, etc.) There will be patients who are registered but leave prior to receiving either a medical evaluation or completing treatment (left without being seen). It is crucial that the ED registration team and whoever is doing the chart capture, coding, and billing agree on the methodology for reconciling ED registrations with billable events. There should also be a mechanism to track and monitor nonbillable patient events. This is a component of transparency that will be very important for anyone being compensated on a productivity basis.

- It is crucial that a complete copy of the chart is available in a reliably timely manner for coding.

- The emergency services group will need to decide which provider gets credit for the patient visit. It is commonplace to transfer care of patients at change of shift, and, consequently, it becomes an issue of who will get credit for that patient visit, the physician who starts the workup or the physician who signs the chart and discharges the patient. If midlevel providers are used within the ED, it is also important to consider whether the work they perform will be incorporated into the productivity model and to what degree it will be incorporated. This becomes important because physician time is required for the supervision being provided and the cosigning of the midlevel provider chart.

This part of due diligence is crucial in order to establish trust and transparency to all of those who will be compensated under a productivity-based system. All providers are cognizant of the fact that there will be certain errors in this process; however, they need to feel assured that there is a process in place to identify errors, correct errors, and complete all adjustments in a fair and timely fashion.

Heading Off Potential Roadblocks

Once your due diligence has been completed and the provider group has acknowledged a level of trust or confidence in the ability to identify billable patients, reconcile credit for each visit, and monitor and correct any errors that occur, the group will be ready to begin the process of designing and implementing the actual productivity compensation system. It's strongly recommended that a work group of the doctors be formed to also include a representative from the billing and coding group to discuss the philosophy and methodology for the system. Some of the mechanics that the group will need to work out include the following questions:

- Is there adequate patient volume 24 hours per day, seven days per week, to ensure that all shifts have the same opportunity for productivity?

- What behaviors (care documentation, patient satisfaction, peer review/risk management, hospital meeting participation/citizenship, etc.) should be linked to compensation and how so?

These philosophic discussions are crucial for the group. They're also crucial for the hospital to ensure that the correct performance behaviors are encouraged. Many hospitals have been reticent to get extensively involved in physician compensation methodologies. However, the productivity-based system allows for alignment of goals and objectives, and therefore, the hospital administration certainly should be in a position to review how the productivity system works.

Note: If the hospital is providing a subsidy to the emergency services group, it certainly has a fiduciary obligation to ensure that those funds are invested in a fashion to create alignment with the board's mission and objectives for organizational performance. Further, once the emergency physician group has agreed to accept a subsidy, it has forfeited its right to maintain full privacy of its compensation methodology and/or conceptual disbursement of funds.

Some of the questions the advisory group will need to deal with include:

- How does the system prevent or deal with chart cherry-picking?

- Does the fast-track compensation need to be adjusted to accommodate enhanced productivity?

- How will midlevel provider revenue be accounted?

Since these issues deal specifically with provider compensation, it's crucial that all physicians have a level of comfort and confidence with the final outcome and have a voice in modifying the compensation methodology over time. Phasing in a productivity compensation system seems beneficial in that some of the fundamental components can be rolled out first, allowing the providers to gain more comfort and confidence with a new methodology before tying in citizenship or other seemingly less-objective performance components.

The group will need to come to grips with what percentage of the total compensation will be productivity driven. This can range from 1%–100% of compensation driven by productivity. Our experience indicates that at least 30% of compensation should be at risk (based on productivity) in order to change behavior. Last, once the methodology and process has been defined, it is recommended that the old system be run in parallel with the new system for at least three to six months. An added benefit to the providers is an agreement to pay the greater of the earnings amount under the old system versus the new system during that tandem period. This is a win for the providers, enhances the provider's focus on the old versus the new system, and allows the individual provider time to understand what types of performance will optimize or increase his or her earning potential. During this tandem period, it is crucial that the necessary tools to enhance performance be available and in place (e.g., coding support, real-time feedback on RVU production, medical director coaching to enhance patient velocity.)

There are huge benefits to productivity-based compensation systems, particularly when they're designed to bring about the following:

- More acutely aligned goals and objectives between the organization and the emergency physician group

- Actively promoted team building and citizenship among the ED team

- Increased patient volume in the ED (an assessment should confirm that the ED plant and staffing resources can accommodate additional volume)

- Transparency, which creates confidence and promotes open participative problem solving within the department

- Increased earnings to the providers

INCENTIVE PLAN PROPOSAL

The following outlines concepts for consideration as the advisory group begins assembling the method and philosophy of the productivity-based plan.

Reward system components:

- A base hourly rate driven by hours worked.

- RVU productivity—40% of total earnings.

- Citizenship—about 4%–5% of total earnings. Activities that count toward the citizenship bonus include:

    - Department meetings attended

    - Other medical staff committee participation

    - In-services, lectures, etc. (documented)

    - Peer review duties

    - Resident teaching (ED attendings only; based on aggregate scores from residents every six months)

Eligibility criteria for the citizenship component:

- Healthcare system computer training completed

- Risk-management protocol competency and patient-satisfaction scripting completed within a specified time period

- Reasonable response time to peer review inquiries (defined as no cases discussed at the department meeting or closed out without provider input and no more than two delayed responses per year)

- Patient-satisfaction scripts for doctors reviewed; improvement coaching presentations reviewed

C H A P T E R

11

Billing, Coding, and Collections

How do emergency medicine groups optimize revenue? There seems to be some question about what services emergency medicine physicians can bill for, what they actually do bill for, and what they actually get reimbursed for. In actuality, the nature of emergency medicine coding and billing is quite straightforward. It centers on ED evaluation and management (E/M) codes 99281–99285, critical care codes 99291 and 99292, and hospital observation codes 99218–99220 and 99234–99236. More than 85% of reimbursement comes through the core ED E/M codes. An emphasis on documentation is crucial to successful revenue optimization. For example, omission of necessary components of the history of presenting illness can result in a potential E/M code 99285 being reimbursed at a 99283 rate, which results in $104 of lost revenue on the Medicare Fee Schedule.

When working with your emergency services group, there should be a shared, coordinated, and highly collaborative focus on accurate and timely documentation. This clearly benefits the hospital from a facility coding perspective and also benefits the emergency services professional group. From the emergency services professional group perspective, it is important that the physicians and midlevel providers understand the documentation guidelines and opportunities to ensure comprehensive and timely documentation.

To provide a benchmark on the facility revenue impact of ED coding, we will use the following figures from, "The Opportunity Loss of Boarding Admitted Patients in the Emergency Department" published in *Academic Emergency Medicine* in 2007, to represent the average facility net revenue:[1]

- An ED visit = $384

- An ED visit that converts into an inpatient admission = $5,432

If your hospital has an ED that has 50,000 visits annually and admits 20% of those visits, you are managing a service line that generates more than $19 million of facility revenue from ED visits (not including all the ancillary revenue) and more than $50 million of inpatient revenue.

It's crucial for the emergency services professional staff members to collaborate on their documentation with the critical care services of the hospital, because it will enable the facility to optimize critical care revenue for inpatient and observation stays. This will also help the organization successfully defend observation stays, particularly as they relate to patients with cardiac events who come to the ED and are held for completion of stress tests or other diagnostic interventions. It is highly recommended that the professional services coding staff coordinate their documentation activities with the facility coding department.

Capturing Missed Revenue

When looking for the most frequently missed revenue opportunities, the professional staff should focus on higher-acuity patient presentations, which can be characterized as a subsequent threat or immediate threat because those areas require the most comprehensive level of documentation. This is where the professional staff and the facility staff (nursing) have opportunity for improvement. High-acuity patients will present a high to extreme risk of morbidity without treatment or a moderate to high risk of mortality without treatment or have a high probability of severe prolonged functional impairment. This is substantiated by any one of the following five indicators:

1. Multiple ancillary studies

2. Special studies (e.g., CT, ultrasound, MRI)

3. IV medications

4. Multiple intramuscular medications

5. Admission or transfer

The history of the present illness (HPI) as documented should contain a chief complaint that clearly reflects the nature of the presenting problem. To substantiate high severity, at least four separate elements within the HPI must be documented. These elements may be location, quality, severity, timing, duration, context, modifying factors, and associated signs and symptoms. When the coders extract these elements from the medical record, they cannot make assumptions or modify the record in any way. The coding can only be substantiated from documentation that conforms to objective facts.

To warrant high severity, the review of systems (ROS) must include positive or pertinent negative responses that are individually documented. For remaining systems, a notation indicating all other systems are negative is permissible.

The past family social history (PFSH) requires documentation of at least one specific item from two of the three history areas. If the physician is unable to obtain a history from the patient or other source, the record should describe the patient's condition or other circumstance that precludes obtaining a history. For example, "History was unobtainable from the patient due to reduced responsiveness. No other source for history was available."

The actual examination to substantiate high severity should include specific negative findings of the organ system. A notation of "abnormal" without elaboration is insufficient. A notation indicating "negative" or "normal" is sufficient to document normal findings.

From these four core assessment areas—HPI, ROS, PFSH, and examination—data are extracted to warrant medical decision-making. Risk factors and diagnostic options complete the medical decision-making tree. Relevant data come in the form of diagnostic services ordered or performed and documentation of the type of service. Everything must be documented, including:

- A review of the diagnostic tests

- Discussions of the diagnostic test with the physician who performed or interpreted the test

- Direct visualization and independent interpretation of an imaging tracing or specimen

- A decision to obtain old records or additional history from another source

- Relevant findings from old records or the additional history source

- Comorbidities and underlying diseases that increase complications, morbidity, or mortality

- Surgical or invasive diagnostic procedures ordered or performed or any referral for such a procedure to be performed on an urgent basis

Critically ill or unstable patients or patients with a high probability of sudden clinically significant or life-threatening deterioration warrant critical status. The treatment criterion may be summarized as requiring constant and full attention at the bedside and involving a high complexity of medical decision-making. Critical care services must be documented based on the amount of time spent. Observation codes may be used when the following clinical criteria are met: an inconclusive diagnosis in which observation may prove admission is unnecessary or may indicate an opportunity for therapeutic resolution, possibly negating the need for admission. The treatment criteria include admission to observation status or an observation treatment plan and the documentation criteria require three key components of the E/M (same requirements, except a past family and social history must be documented). The admitting physician must date and time the order, and discharge documentation must be present.

The emergency services group should be knowledgeable about coding requirements; the emergency services coding professionals should supply routinely conducted audit results substantiating billing codes used; and the emergency services group should coordinate all training activities with the facility coders. Additionally, the emergency services group should routinely review documentation to ensure appropriateness and compliance with respective standards. Nursing staff members should be intimately involved in any recommended changes to forms that enhance nursing documentation, as well as physician documentation. The medical records department and/or health information management department should also be involved to review any changes from a coding and documentation compliance perspective.

NONPHYSICIAN PRACTITIONERS

The following are rules regarding the use of nonphysician practitioners—such as physician assistants or nurse practitioners—and scribes.

The face-to-face rule

- If the E/M of a patient is shared between a physician and a midlevel provider from the same group practice and the physician provides any face-to-face portion of the E/M encounter with the patient, the service may be billed under the physician's unique physician identification number (UPIN).

- If there was no face-to-face encounter between the patient and the physician (e.g., even if the physician participated in the service only by reviewing the patient's medical record), then the service may only be billed under the midlevel practitioner's UPIN.

- Payment will be made at the appropriate physician fee schedule rate based on the UPIN entered on the claim. This impacts the reimbursement levels for the professional service group, and, certainly, if midlevel providers are not employed by the emergency services group, this may significantly impact reimbursement.

Scribe rules

- Each entry into the medical record made by a medical scribe may only be made at the direction of the ED physician

- The entry should include the date and time of the entry and should contain language similar to "written by [name of scribe], acting as scribe for Dr. [Smith]"

Cash on the Line

The physician voluntary reporting program (pay for performance)—the Tax Relief and Health Care Act of 2006 (H.R. 6111), which stops the 5.1% reduction in Medicare payment and provides for an additional 1.5% increase—began in July 2007 for physicians who agree to report quality-of-care data to the government. The current ED measures being reviewed under pay for performance include:

- Receiving aspirin and a beta-blocker at arrival for acute myocardial infarction (AMI)

- EKG performed for nontraumatic chest pain

- Thrombolytic therapy ordered within 20 minutes of an EKG performed for AMI

- Care coordination for percutaneous coronary intervention for AMI

- EKG performed for syncopy

- Vital signs checked for pneumonia

- Assessment for oxygen saturation for pneumonia

- Assessment for mental status for pneumonia

- Empiric antibiotic for pneumonia

Collection of these data in a fashion that demonstrates the degree of compliance will be important for reporting purposes for pay for performance.

Due to the limited E/M codes used by emergency services physicians and midlevel providers, the fact that emergency medicine professionals provide services under the guidelines of the Emergency Medical Treatment and Active Labor Act of 1986 (treat all comers), and compared to other physicians' specialties in the hospital, emergency service physicians tend to receive a lower percentage of charges in reimbursement, so documentation is imperative to the success of your emergency physician group. Any medical group affiliated with the hospital or being contemplated should be able to thoroughly defend its active documentation training process and coding compliance review process and want to fully engage with the facility's coding staff to heighten revenue optimization.

Reference

1. Falvo, T., Grove, L., Stachura, R., Vega, D., Stike, R., Schlenker, M., and Zirkin, W. 2007. "The Opportunity Loss of Boarding Admitted Patients in the Emergency Department." *Academic Emergency Medicine* 14(4): 332–337.

The Business Case

Ask anyone working in healthcare what our chief task is, and the answer is likely to be serving patients and communities. This is true enough. However, the idea of service has an important implication. A service business means we compete for customers and resources. Improving flow has twin purposes: to provide better service and to attain financial goals.

Teaming those two components—not pitting them against each other—will get your hospital system across the finish line. If the service we provide (in business terms, a product) is poor, then our business will decline. And if our business falls off, we may be unable to provide service to our patients. To provide better service, we need to follow sound business principles.

The need is even more pressing today than it was in the recent past. Historians will no doubt record 2008 and 2009 as the years an extraordinary global financial crisis invaded our lives. Bankruptcies, foreclosures, tight credit, tumbling stock prices, rising unemployment, and evaporating 401(k)s were reported hourly.

On top of the economic crisis, the pay-for-performance model has increasingly come into play. Many patients have choices about where they can get their healthcare, and they're not reluctant to exercise those choices. To attract patients' business, healthcare systems increasingly will have to find ways to satisfy customer expectations for service. If ever there was a time to define and defend the business case for improving patient flow, it is now.

When you consider your current financial pressures, the economic benefits of improving flow create their own convincing argument: increased revenues, reduced costs and waste, and improved service, safety, and satisfaction. Taking steps to enhance patient flow can empower administrators and medical directors to effectively address shrinking margins and increased competition. The business case for hardwiring patient flow is compelling.

Building the Business Case

When building the business case for improving flow, you need to relate such improvement to revenue. In simple terms, improved patient flow leads to increased capacity, increased ED revenue, and increased hospital revenue. When you make the case effectively, the system administration will support the project to improve flow. The approach should be businesslike. For example:

- Develop a business plan complete with objectives, anticipated costs, and expected revenues

- Explain the metrics you will use to determine the success of your improvement plan

- Focus on clinical excellence, operational quality and effectiveness, customer satisfaction, and sound financial management

One of the fundamentals of successful ED management is teamwork. Hiring the right people and building an effective team leads to well-flowing operations and staff satisfaction. From a business perspective, you can provide some concrete projections in regard to the benefits of a high-performance team. For starters, determine what your break-even points for personnel costs are, using the following factors:

- Cost per hour of physician staffing

- Cost per hour of nursing staffing

- Cost of overtime (hours of overtime multiplied by staffing costs per hour equals overtime costs per day [or week, month, or year])

- Cost of extra physician coverage and overtime

- Cost of extra nursing coverage and overtime

Then, illustrate how having an effective team translates into financial terms. Two useful concepts in business management are net patient revenue (NPR) and contribution margin (CM).

For the purposes of this discussion, we will define NPR as the average expected payment for a patient service. Once the direct expenses that are incurred to deliver the respective service are subtracted from the NPR, the resultant difference is the CM.

In healthcare, the NPR comes from patient visits and related procedures, and the costs represent expenses incurred in providing these services. Another concept we'll use later in this chapter is patient velocity (PV), which is a calculation of the number of patient visits divided by the clinical hours required to render those visits.

Examples

To convey the financial implications of a stable, satisfied workforce, here are two examples. The first shows the costs of high turnover, specifically what hiring a new physician might cost, and illustrates the money saved by avoiding recruitment costs.

Recruiting costs:

- Recruiting fee—$20,000

- Ancillary costs (interviewing travel and entertainment expenses)—$5,000

- Signing bonus—$5,000–$10,000

- Moving expenses—$2,500–$10,000

- Time, effort, energy—unmeasured but true costs

- Total recruiting costs = $40,000

Assimilation costs:

- Productivity (e.g., six months at a PV of less than one patient per hour [or less than 0.5 or 0.25] multiplied by NPR per patient equals decrease in patient flow dollars—an opportunity cost)

- Teamwork building

You can see that the cost to a system of recruiting a new physician can be substantial. Compounding this recruitment cost are associated costs—for example, the added stress imposed on other team members making up for the current shortage (potential burnout). Staff satisfaction decreases during staff shortage periods that extend either indefinitely or beyond four to six months. This can be particularly challenging, because the average time period from identifying the need to having the new physician working a schedule is nine months or longer for a physician.

This next example illustrates the potential revenues associated with retaining effective and satisfied, stable staff members in a well-flowing operation:

- The average NPR (facility fee) for an ED visit is $400

- With a moderate flow-improvement initiative successfully implemented, PV can increase from 1.75 to 2

- $1.75 \times \$400 = \$700$ of hourly NPR; $2 \times \$400 = \$800$ of hourly NPR

- Every 0.25 increase in a physician's PV equals a $100 hourly increase in NPR

- Every one-hour decrease in physician staffing costs equals $150 in savings

- Every one-hour change in physician coverage per day equals a direct expense reduction of $54,750 per year or a CM improvement of almost $55,000

A clinically excellent, effective team in a well-flowing operation also helps mitigate the risks of medical malpractice. The potential savings of reducing those risks can be substantial.

Operational Quality and Effectiveness

Readers of a certain age probably remember the sign that used to be outside every McDonald's® restaurant that gave the total number of customers served by the chain. This statistic wasn't just a marketing gimmick. It reflected the principle well known by fast-food restaurants: The faster tables turn over, the more customers are served, and the more profits increase. For owners of restaurants, financial gain is indicated more by table turnovers than by the number of tables occupied at any given time.

The same principle applies to healthcare. The best way to increase profit is to serve more customers. For EDs, serving more customers equates to improving through-put so that PV increases, with PV measuring the number of patients seen (or treated or processed) per hour. For the hospital as a whole, serving more customers means increasing the number of bed turns. Figure 12.1 offers some concrete ways of calculating how increasing the number of bed turns can impact your system.

FIGURE 12.1

INCREASING BED TURNS

Number of patients seen per bed per day equals the number of hours per day (in the ED, postanesthesia care unit, or ICU) or days per year (inpatients) a bed is available divided by the average throughput time per bedded patient. For example, if:

- ED length of stay (LOS) equals four hours, then each bed serves six patients per day

- Hospital LOS equals 4.5 days, then each bed serves 81 patients per year (365 / 4.5 = 81)

To quantify the impact of throughput reduction through improving flow, consider the example of reducing throughput time by 11% per bed, which equals improvement of hospital LOS from 4.5 to four days. The impact of this improvement translates to:

- 91.25 patients per bed per year or 10.25 additional patients treated

- $76,875 NPR annually per bed, at an average NPR of $7,500 per admission

- $3,843,750 annual NPR improvement (considering that this average hospital LOS improvement is experienced in 50 beds representing the medical floors)

Again, a very modest increase has a dramatic effect, as you can see from this calculation of the impact of admitting one more patient each day through the ED:

- 20 admissions per day × $7,500 per admission on average = $54,750,000 per year NPR

- 21 admissions per day × $7,500 per admission on average = $57,487,500 per year NPR

- 1 more admission per day = $2,737,500 per year additional NPR for your system

---

When you make the business case for improving flow, you should also illustrate the flip side of increasing admissions and bed turns—what we call opportunity cost. That cost is the potential revenue you lose through lost admissions, such as walkaways and diversions. Walkaways fall into several categories, generally seen in the ED. Those categories comprise patients who leave without being seen, leave without being treated, or leave against medical advice, without completing recommended treatment. The following is a calculation of the opportunity costs of walkaways:

- NPR for physician services (e.g., $100 per patient) × the number of patients leaving per year = the opportunity cost per year for physician services

- NPR for hospital services (e.g., $400 per patient) × the number of patients leaving per year = the opportunity cost per year for the hospital

- NPR for an admitted patient (e.g., $7,500) × the number of patients leaving per year × the admission percentage = the opportunity cost per year for the hospital

- Using a conservative estimate for lost admissions of 5% of walkaway patients, the opportunity cost in the contribution margin per patient for admissions (e.g., $7,500) × the number of patients not seen × 5% = the potential revenue from lost admissions

Using this formula with the example amounts for various services, a hospital system with an ED averaging 50,000 patient visits per year would realize $50,000 in new physician revenue without any increased overhead if it reduced the number of walkaways by 1%. Again this is $50,000 in new revenue without any increased overhead. Similarly, the system would realize $387,500 in new NPR for that 1% reduction. A seemingly modest 1% change can yield significant financial results.

Diversions to other hospitals because of limited capacity entail similar opportunity costs of lost revenue. Continuing with the 50,000 annual visit ED example, on average six patients per hour are being treated, and one of those six gets admitted each hour (16% admission rate). Using our average figure from earlier of $7,500 NPR from an admitted patient, 6 visits × $400 NPR + 1 admission × $7,500 lost NPR = $9,900 lost NPR per hour of diversion.

Each hour your ED is on diversion, you are turning away almost $10,000 of NPR. If that isn't enough to make your chief financial officer groan loudly, combine the amount of direct expenses you are still paying for staff members to treat the patients you are diverting. You can see the impact a single hour makes when you calculate the cumulative amount of lost revenue per hour of diversion based on your system's average number of diversions. Additional factors that go into calculating opportunity costs are the labor hours spent diverting and the cost of processing lost patients within the ED.

A different type of opportunity cost results from the burden of boarding. If you have inpatients taking up outpatient beds in the ED or operating room, your system is losing potential revenue from the blocked capacity. Think of jets sitting in a queue on a runway awaiting takeoff. The flight for Atlanta is ready to go, but it can't leave until the flight for Orlando takes off. But that one can't leave until the flight for Boston gets clearance, and so on. Using the average figures for your system, you can calculate what this opportunity cost is per day, per month, and per year.

Quality is an integral factor when working to improve flow for operational effectiveness as well. Simply working to increase PV and bed turns to make money is not the goal. The goal is working to improve flow, which leads to increased PV and bed turns and, ultimately, more revenue in conjunction with increased quality of service and shorter stays. A restaurant that concentrates solely on turning tables as quickly as possible and neglects the quality of its food and service won't stay in business long.

Customer Satisfaction

Improving flow in an ED and hospital system as a whole results in smoother processes that lead to increased PV but also better service and shorter stays. Patients aren't going to mind being turned out of bed, so to speak, more quickly if they're receiving high-quality care and attention and being treated efficiently. The good thing about improving patient flow is that the various components affected are interconnected and improving one improves the others as well. When your initiatives work to improve flow, you improve throughput time, resulting in more satisfied patients. Improved patient satisfaction has two results: A happy patient is more likely to return to the hospital for services again and more likely to recommend the hospital to friends, relatives, and associates. Conversely, poor service is an opportunity cost: the organization loses repeat patronage and prospective business from others through word-of-mouth communication from dissatisfied patients.

The benefits of improved flow in regard to customer service can be seen as an increase in visits and a decrease in complaints. Both lead to increased inpatient and outpatient velocity. When handling patient complaints, the organization is spending money (in processing costs and staffing time) that could be saved in a system with better flow.

Sound Financial Management

Improving patient flow involves several components of effective business management: managing costs; increasing PV and NPR per patient; handling documentation, coding, and billing more efficiently; and dealing with "chart stragglers." Several innovative techniques have proven beneficial in implementing better management, such as:

- Template charts

- Scribes

- A checkout register

- Discounts offered for on-site processing of patient bills

- On-site credit card processing

Let's take a look at using scribes, for example. Scribes are typically college students who document patients' medical treatment for nurses or physicians. Healthcare organizations need to use resources effectively, which means having physicians perform duties only they can do. Using scribes fulfills this principle and frees nurses and doctors to concentrate on their core responsibilities. Scribes should not be difficult to recruit, either. What do you think the average college student would prefer: flipping burgers or maintaining charts?

The following are three reasons for allowing scribes to document:

1. Improved chart legibility, which will benefit not only current medical personnel who read the charts but also anyone who may need to read them in the future.

2. Increased ED efficiency. Staff members can see more patients, and the ED can decrease the number of walkaways or length of time spent on diversion. Scribes can also help track labs and x-rays more effectively.

3. Accurate documentation of the medical record. Reducing incorrect or incomplete documentation increases hospital reimbursement levels. For example, one hospital recovered its investment in scribes in two months and subsequently hired scribes for physician assistants as well.

Using scribes can be a sound business practice that improves flow, alleviates workloads of highly stretched nursing teams, and, in so doing, increases staff satisfaction. The components in the ED and the hospital as a whole are extremely interrelated. Improve one and you're likely to improve others as well.

Benefits of using scribes: a metric-driven analysis

Hospital A is a rural North Carolina community facility, and its ED has 31,000 annual visits. BestPractices began staffing the ED in November 2005. The ED was staffed with single physician coverage and a midlevel provider staffing a fast track 10 hours per day. The fast track was frequently closed so the midlevel provider could assist the physician in the main ED. Scribes were hired as part of the ED team to help the physicians more efficiently treat patients in the main emergency room, assist during the installation of an electronic health record, and provide support to the physician, minimizing the need to close the fast track.

What we did

A scribe program was implemented with 250 hours of scribe coverage per week at an hourly rate of approximately $10. The cost per month for the scribes was $11,000. The physicians contributed 50% of the expense to subsidize the scribe program, with the management service company providing the additional 50%.

Figure 12.2 demonstrates down-code percentages before and after the use of scribes, turnaround times, and actual patient velocity by providers. The table also summarizes monthly and per-visit costs and benefits of the scribe program.

FIGURE 12.2

FINANCIAL BENEFITS OF USING SCRIBES

	Pre-scribe	Post-scribe
Doctor A		
LOS	225	200
Down-codes	7.60%	2.40%
PV	2.1	2.4
Doctor B		
LOS	210	190
Down-codes	6.25%	1.85%
PV	2.2	2.5

	Monthly	Per visit
Monthly patient visits	2,583	—
Monthly cost of scribes	$7,280.00	$2.82
Monthly improvement		
Cost of patients who left without being seen (LWBS)	$7,750.00	$3
Down-codes	$5,812.50	$2.25
Net improvement		$2.43

 The Hospital Executive's Guide to Emergency Department Management

Our findings and recommendations

The program effectively assisted physicians in improving documentation (50% down-code reduction), decreasing LOS, and improving patient velocity. The improvement in LOS also enabled a reduction of 3% of patients who LWBS. The physicians demonstrated ownership of the program and were very involved in upgrading the scribes' skill sets. Our recommendations included the following:

- Physicians should financially contribute to subsidize the scribe program to enhance ownership

- Metrics (LOS, down-codes, PV, LWBS) should be well understood and doctor-specific in order to demonstrate improvement

- Physicians should have at least 30% of their compensation based on relative value unit production in order to enhance their commitment to improvement

- A lead scribe who orients and monitors performance should be involved in managing the scribe program

Proposal to front-load patient care and service with nursing, physician, and clinical support deployed in the new triage/treatment area

Suburban Midwest Community Hospital—June 2009

The situation

Effective May 1, 2009, BestPractices ceased staffing triage with midlevel providers. The nursing staff assumed triage responsibility and scheduled RNs to perform this function. BestPractices and the ED nursing staff wanted to front-load patient care and service through a clinician in the triage program. This involved reworking patient flow by streamlining, front-loading, and segmenting patient intake, assessment, and care at the patient's point of entry into the ED. The aim was to reduce length of stay (LOS), increase patient satisfaction, increase medical staff satisfaction, and reduce process redundancy. The improved segmentation process began in May to fine-tune all aspects of this staffing change prior to the execution of the second phase of an ED renovation— patient care addition—taking place in September 2009.

The background

Emergency services was beginning the second phase of its ED renovation, which meant there would be a relocation of, and significant downsizing of, the patient entrance, waiting area, and triage area. The relocation of the entrance, waiting, and triage areas would also result in 75 more yards of hallway before entering the ED patient-treatment area from the entrance, waiting, and triage areas. The ED was committed to sustaining and enhancing patient and medical staff satisfaction and patient safety during phase II and phase III of the ED renovation.

CASE STUDY	**Proposal to front-load patient care and service with nursing, physician, and clinical support deployed in the new triage/treatment area (cont.)**

What we did

Emergency management services have an opportunity to reconfigure all the front-end processes for patient flow. By enhancing triage, using ATPs more consistently, and targeting its use of physicians in the fast track, the ED could favorably impact the goals listed earlier and help improve satisfaction. More importantly, placing a physician in the triage or front-door area at peak patient arrival times is responsible resource allocation to ensure patient safety during a significant change in patient flow and it heightens the likelihood of achieving the other goals listed.

The results

BestPractices and the hospital's ED nursing leadership have developed a rapid intervention and treatment zone—an advanced triage unit (ATU) program—that enhances the front-end assessment and treatment services by using a physician eight hours per day in the new triage area. BestPractices will reallocate the 11-hour-per-day main room mid-level provider resources toward funding this project and request that the hospital fund additional per month cost if necessary. There are metrics to carefully measure the volume treated and released from the ATU, medical staff satisfaction, and door-to-doctor time. Reports will be presented within two months of the program initiation and each month thereafter.

CASE STUDY — Proposal to front-load patient care and service with nursing, physician, and clinical support deployed in the new triage/treatment area (cont.)

FIGURE 12.3

THE BUSINESS CASE

Metric	Proposition	Benefit	Cost
Left without being seen (LWBS)	During a challenging front-door relocation, the ATU investment will reduce the potential of an increase in LWBS	Each 1% of LWBS costs NCH $95,000 of facility revenue*	$42,916 (50% born by BestPractices) or $21,458 to NCH
Improved volume	Implementation of the ATU serves to market/promote the NCH emergency services and increase volume	Each 2.5% increase in volume generates $237,500 new facility revenue**	$42,916 (50% born by BestPractices) or $21,458 to NCH (same as above—no new monies)
Improved patient satisfaction	Implementation of the ATU reduces door-to-doctor time and overall treat-and-release LOS	See above for reduced LWBS and improved volume	

* 5,000 monthly visits x 1% = 50 visits; 30% admission rate x 50 = 15 x $5,432 revenue/admission = $81,000 + 70% x 50 visits = 35 x $384 outpatient ED facility revenue = $14,000.

** Same revenue calculations as above times 2.5.

 The Hospital Executive's Guide to Emergency Department Management

ED staffing provider change—90-day notice

The situation

- A central Illinois ED with 24,000 annual visits was staffed by a contracted ED management company for three years

- The hospital was heavily subsidizing the management company, and the management company was achieving a suboptimal financial contribution margin from services provided

- Recruitment efforts had been suboptimal

- A trial of midlevel providers in the ED was unsuccessful

The background

Two physicians had assumed the medical director role during the first three years of the management staffing company's tenure. Both made some progress; however, recruitment was unsuccessful. Other efforts to fully staff the ED were also unsuccessful (using midlevel providers, reconfiguring staff hours, etc.).

Another hospital in town competed for emergency medicine clinicians. In addition, the community, which was thought to be an attractive recruitment site, proved exceedingly difficult to recruit new emergency medicine clinicians.

The management staffing company and hospital administration met to consider alternatives, such as:

CASE STUDY

ED staffing provider change—90-day notice (cont.)

- Spin the practice into an independently governed and managed group to take over the exclusive-service agreement

- Pursue the hospital's parent company to take over staffing the ED

- Consider a bid from a local independent group

- Choose not to pursue another staffing company

What we did

After a 30-day evaluation period, multiple meetings, and a very careful analysis of advantages and disadvantages, a transition was made between the management staffing company and a newly formed local independent group. This newly formed group was composed of physicians staffing the competitor ED group and existing physicians employed by the management company. The corporate structure, negotiation with the hospital, and formulation of an exclusive service agreement was achieved in 45 days, allowing for a transition on September 1, 2007.

Our findings and conclusions

- The management service company had formed a sound, candid relationship with the client and wanted to find the best service delivery outcome for the client organization.

CASE
STUDY

ED staffing provider change—90-day notice (cont.)

- The client secured a local independent group composed of local physicians committed to the central Illinois community and ensured all subsidy would be delivered to that home-team group.

- The management staffing company achieved a client whose needs were met successfully, a satisfied medical staff, and a transition out of a staffing engagement that did not meet financial expectations. The hospital remains a good reference for the management service company.

Candid, transparent involvement by a management service provider and administration and hospital medical staff is essential for identifying and contemplating alternative arrangements to provide emergency services staffing.

CASE STUDY

Streamlining patient flow by redesigning the intake area

The situation

A large hospital in suburban Chicago needed to streamline patient flow. Construction and redesign of the intake area was proposed. Although construction presented challenges to capacity, staffing, and service, it would ultimately deliver a new patient-care addition for inpatient utilization and a modernized ED.

Several pieces had to be in place prior to a successful implementation, such as:

- Gaining organizational support

- Establishing triage champions

- Creating a data-driven design

- Implementing patient segmentation

What we did

Gained organizational support

It became clear that a redesign of the patient intake process (triage) would be necessary. It was decided that this was our opportunity for improvement, and it was important to communicate this to the organization. Top-level support during any process-improvement project lends a level of importance to the project. It also ensures that there is appropriate alignment with the organization's initiatives. We were able to effectively communicate the potential impact that the phased reconstruction could have on the organization. The best means to prevent any compromises in quality of care, patient safety, patient satisfaction, and potential loss of business would be to implement a patient-intake team

The Hospital Executive's Guide to Emergency Department Management

Streamlining patient flow by redesigning the intake area (cont.)

termed the advanced triage unit (ATU). These elements were mutually important, and we had the full support of hospital leadership.

Established triage champions

A team of providers, recognized as either strong performers or having a strong interest in participating, was assembled. The team consisted of a physician, nursing representation from each shift, medical techs, staff members from phlebotomy and registration, and radiology techs. This group served as the core team for facilitating change. The initial practical elements for the team were flow-charting the current patient intake process and identifying inefficient aspects within the process.

Used data-driven design

In developing our process for improving patient flow, an important step was to fully understand which patients would potentially utilize the service (demand). It was equally important to know how many providers and beds (capacity) were necessary to provide the service. This was accomplished by analyzing patient-arrival data over a period and determining how many patients present to the ED per hour.

It was determined that demand was approximately seven patients per hour. Of the seven patients who present, we needed to determine who would be processed through the ATU. It is known that two patients per hour are low acuity (acuity index [AI] Level 4 and 5). This population would primarily be treated and dispositioned by the ATU. The remaining five patients per hour are of moderate acuity (AI Level 3). The ability to treat and release 20% of that patient population from the ATU would provide additional capacity in our main patient care area.

Streamlining patient flow by
redesigning the intake area (cont.)

Established patient segmentation

An appropriate alignment of resources with the services required by the patient is a key aspect of process improvement. It was helpful to have a prior AI classification. The AI enabled us to segment our patient care streams based on acuity and design processes around those patients who required little intervention. (See Figures 12.4 and 12.5.)

We were able to take advantage of the space adjacent to the waiting area to serve as a an area for waiting for results. We utilized a tracking board to follow patients throughout the area. The combination of the results waiting area and the tracking board provided some additional capacity, creating a virtual bed.

FIGURE 12.4

PATIENT SEGMENTATION

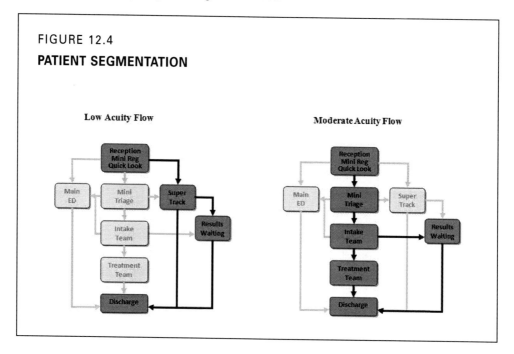

Streamlining patient flow by redesigning the intake area (cont.)

FIGURE 12.5

STREAMLINED FRONT-END ED PATIENT FLOW

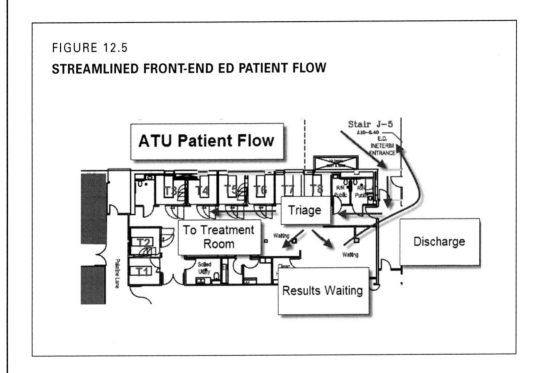

CASE STUDY

Streamlining patient flow by redesigning the intake area (cont.)

Our findings and conclusions

We gathered data during our first three weeks of operation. The numbers of patients that left without being seen or desired to leave against medical advice were both less than 1%. As there are AI Level 3, 4, and 5 patients seen in the ATU, the data reflected the mixture of this patient population. The average LOS for patients treated and released by the ATU was less than two hours, whereas it is three hours in other areas of the department.

What was not captured in the data but provided tremendous benefit to the department were the numerous patients that were evaluated and had their care initiated in the ATU. These patients consistently had a decreased LOS in comparison to similar patients in the department. The patient care experience in the ATU has been overwhelmingly positive.

Implementing a patient-intake team with a physician at the initial point of care was a welcomed addition to emergency services at our institution. The fortuitous design has assisted in weathering the higher volumes of a seasonal surge. There was no significant loss of business during this period of construction. This process improvement has enabled the ED to ensure patient safety, provide quality care, and maintain a high level of patient satisfaction.